Dr. Thomas L. Stone attended our dental health seminar in Chicago. When asked why a medical doctor would attend a dental seminar, Dr. Stone said, **"I know you dentists are killing my patients, I just want to find out how you are doing it."**

Dr. Stone's statement encouraged me to write this book.

Douglas L. Cook, D.D.S. graduated from Marquette School of Dentistry in 1954. Two years as a dentist in Germany honed his skills working on military service men and women. Returning to his home in Wisconsin, he started a practice in 1956.

He is a past member of the American Dental Association, Wisconsin Dental Association, Marinette Oconto County Dental Society, Wisconsin Dental Society of Anesthesiology, American Academy of Biological Dentistry, Center for Chinese Medicine, International Academy of Oral Medicine and Toxicology, and Holistic Dental Association.

He has attended three seminars by Dr. Reinhold Voll, MD, on Electro Acupuncture, now known as Computerized Electro-dermal Screening. He has also taken continuing education courses on health problems related to the oral cavity, an area often overlooked in health exams.

Dr. Cook has presented over 20 seminars on dental materials and Computerized Electro-dermal screening, in Asia, Mexico, Australia, and Canada, as well as in the United States.

Dr. Cook's fifty-five years in dentistry have shown him that there is a NEED to help patients suffering from illnesses directly related to the oral cavity.

RESCUED BY MY DENTIST

NEW SOLUTIONS TO A HEALTH CRISIS

By

Douglas L. Cook, D.D.S., S.C.

Order this book online at www.trafford.com
or email orders@trafford.com

Most Trafford titles are also available at major online book retailers.

Print information available on the last page.

ISBN: 978-1-4251-7091-2 (sc)
ISBN: 978-1-4269-7838-8 (e)

Trafford rev. 08/19/2021

www.trafford.com

North America & international
toll-free: 844-688-6899 (USA & Canada)
fax: 812 355 4082

Acknowledgements

Fifty-five years of practicing dentistry and consulting with both professionals and patients have made this book possible. Naming everyone would go far beyond these page's, however there are some key people I want to acknowledge. First and foremost is my father, who said "go be a dentist." Dr. Reinhold Voll, M.D., gave me my start in energy dentistry and medicine. Dr. Thomas L. Stone, M.D., taught me the effects of dental materials on patient's health and saved my life on two occasions with his skills and knowledge. Dr. Vincent Speckhart, M.D., opened another door to the influence of dental materials on the survival of patients. I thank all of you.

The patients whose case histories are told throughout this book encouraged me to tell their story so that all health professionals can see another way to health through the oral cavity.

Organizations such as the International Academy of Oral Medicine and Toxicology, The Holistic Dental Association, The Academy of Biological Dentistry and Medicine, with DAMS (Dental Amalgam Mercury Solutions) and Consumers for Dental Choice are all dedicated to making a difference in dentistry and their patients. Each generously offered the knowledge and techniques that helped me to see the way to help many.

A thank you goes to my assistants, Melissa and Michele, my computer helpers. Thank you to Amber, my sister, and Louann Vertrees of AZProofreader, for all their help in proofreading and suggestions. Another thank you goes to Cheri Dorr of Dorr Design Associates, Inc. for the beautiful layouts and book cover design.

Contents

Forward:

I have known Dr. Doug Cook since 1996 when I met him during the coldest winter in Chicago. Dr. Cook was sponsoring a Conference on Energy in Medicine and Dentistry. I was one of the few medical doctors who attended to find out "how dentists are killing my patients" as eloquently stated by Tom Stone, MD.

Too many complex medical problems are originated by dental problems and from the dental treatment done by dentists. Most medical doctors don't understand the relationship between the body/tooth connections. They continue looking elsewhere for the cause of the problems, when most common chronic illnesses come from right under their patient's nose, the oral cavity and the teeth.

I've been practicing Internal Medicine for over 20 years. I didn't realize the magnitude of the influence of the oral cavity and dental pathology as the culprits of medical problems until I attended Dr. Cook's conference. Dental problems are associated with arthritis, chronic pain and inflammations, heart disease and heart attack, cancer, headaches, fatigue, insomnia, and kidney disorder, just to name a few disorders.

Actually, medical schools teach about dental related medical conditions like endocarditis, arthritis, and nephritis. However, we didn't have the reliable tools to measure and evaluate the connections between the teeth and the body. Chapters 7 through 22 introduce you to Computerized Electro-Dermal Screening (CEDS) to perform an "acupuncture meridian assessment."

I was fortunate to be introduced to CEDS by Dr. Cook at that Energy Medicine conference for dentists. I was skeptical at first. I came back for another conference on CEDS. My skepticism was transformed into a totally new way of looking at the human body as a form of meridians and energy fields. It changed my practice of medicine forever. Practicing medicine became fun. Patients got well.

Medicine made sense as I learned more about illness by studying dentistry.

Dr. Cook takes the reader into a new kind of dentistry, that of energy medicine. The chapters cover detailed information on the dangers of root canals, amalgams and other dental materials, unrecognized cavitations, implants, metal oxides incompatibilities, denture materials and many more commonly over looked problems caused by dentists.

This book is written for dentists, medical professionals and for the general public. For those people suffering from seemingly incurable medical conditions, this book may give you new hope. Share this book with your dentist and your medical doctors.

This book is the accumulated knowledge of over 50 years of Dr. Cook's clinical experience. Including the wisdom and knowledge of his father, that makes one hundred years of dentistry experience. Some of the topics, especially those on CEDS and energetic relationships, might be controversial or hard to grasp. However, don't let that get in your way of discovering your own healing process.

The results are the ultimate criteria for success. Dr. Cook wrote this book because of his results. I've been personally honored to see the results for myself when knowledge of energy medicine is applied to the tooth and body connection.

Read this book with an open mind and you will be rewarded with Dr. Cook's inspirational writing through incredible case studies. Dr. Cook will take you to a new energetic dentistry by rescuing and curing incurable patients. Dr. Tom Stone was correct when he said, "I know you dentists are killing my patients. I just want to find out how you are doing it."

Simon M. Yu, M.D.

Preface

In my early years, the dental chair and I became great friends. The good part of that was that my father, Irving Cook, being a dentist, saved my teeth from the ravages of decay; the bad part is that all of my amalgam fillings contained 50% mercury. We didn't realize at the time that the mercury from my fillings, along with food allergies, were the cause of my sore throats, sinus infections, stomach aches, sleepless nights, tonsillitis and eye problems. In addition, my mother knew very little about healthy eating. We ate anything with sugar on it, through it, over it or under it. As a result, I had had thirty-seven mercury amalgam fillings placed in my teeth.

My father, after surviving four heart attacks, began a push to find a better way to health than conventional medical treatments. It was Dr. Melvin Page of St Petersburg, Florida, who set a bottle of minerals in front of my father and said to him, "take these the rest of your life". Dr. Page knew the soil in this country had become seriously depleted of minerals, thus short-changing our food supply and leaving the total population in worse health. After I returned from my military tour as a dentist in 1956, my father put me on the Body Chemistry Balancing program that had been formulated by Dr. Page. The example of my father, along with Dr. Page's s nutritional advice, put me on a personal path to better health.

It would not be until 1979 that I understood that mercury "silver amalgam" fillings play a serious role in my health problems and in most health problems. My personal path gave rise to a journey of change in my professional practice; there would be a number of important teachers and mentors. Dr. Ed Arana, D.D.S., founder of the American Academy of Biological Dentistry, brought brilliant minds to his seminars on total health, helping to connect the mouth to the rest of the body.

After learning how to do ear acupuncture for pain control, I sought out advanced study with Dr. Reinhold Voll, from

Germany. Dr. Voll's famous statement that "80 to 90 percent of systemic problems are caused, or influenced by the oral cavity, tonsils, and sinuses," still holds true today. Dr. Voll's invention, EAV (Electro-acupuncture by Voll), sometimes called electro-dermal screening, involves the use of conductance points (acupuncture points) on the hands and feet to allow exploration of the entire meridian-energy system. Dr. Andrew Landerman, D.D.S., led me through the important steps of EAV and the relationship of teeth to the organ and tissue systems of the body. Both Dr. Landerman and another dentist, Dr. Christian, taught me that the metal oxides, commonly used in composite fillings, are incompatible with the patient.

Dr. Harold Kristal, D.D.S., made important presentations about nutrition and basic body chemistry; he pointed out how deficiencies are able to cause poor health. Dr. David Eggelston D.D.S., as well as Dr. Kristal, researched the detrimental effects of metals on the immune system. Both Dr. Ralph Turk, D.D.S. and Dr. Krammer, D.D.S., gave outstanding lectures on the harmful effects of high speed dental drilling; following their lectures, I changed from high to low speed drilling in my dental practice, allowing me to better save my patient's teeth. Both of these dentists also pointed out how a wide variety of symptoms and adverse health effects are readily produced by the electrical effects of metal fillings and other metal dental materials in our mouths. The late Dr. Thomas Stone, M.D., would become an important friend and collaborator. I still remember how he startled the dentists at the seminar when he told us why he was there: "I know you dentists are killing my patients, I just want to find out *how* you are doing it." He drove home the importance of dental effects on patients' health.

Other important influences came later in my journey. Dr. Vincent Speckhart, M.D., was an oncologist who investigated the use of EAV extensively. His use of both homeopathy and dental revision to aid his patient's and enhanced their ability to overcome cancer. Removal of root canalled teeth, infected teeth, jawbone cavitations, dental metals of all kind and recovery from pesticide poisoning all became important elements of Dr. Speckhart's treatment protocols. His 80% success rate for cancer patient recovery pointed out the importance of biological dentistry as a key to survival and recovery.

Dr. Boyd Haley, Ph.D., Professor of Chemistry at the University of Kentucky became a pioneer in the measurement of the toxicity of biopsied teeth and jawbone material. Dr. Haley asserted that all root canal treated teeth are infected to some extent and that most of them test as being toxic or even "extremely toxic." Dr. Haley also developed the TOPAS and the Halitox test as a quick chair-side test for the dentist to use to determine the degree of bacterial and protein toxicity in the fluid sample taken from root canal treated teeth or next to infected, dying teeth. Dr. Haley's lab tests on jawbone biopsies also have revealed that the material in the dead-bone areas of jawbone cavitations always "contain toxic material."

Dr. Boyd Haley, Dr. Vincent Speckhart, and the others have contributed to changing patient's health by changing the practice of dentistry. All of these professionals have added to my ability to protect my patient's health and improve their recovery from illnesses. This book describes my own views and what I regard as best dental practices. These principles, and the patient stories that illustrate them, are interwoven with the teachings and the important influences from my entire career.

I believe that ALL health professional schools need a course in dental health, detailing the effect of the oral cavity on the entire health of the patient. Having a good understanding of the far-reaching influence of metals, incompatible composites, denture plastics, root canals and jawbone infections/cavitations would save millions of dollars in health care costs.

Dentistry makes a difference.

Introduction

DAMS is the major education and support group in America for dental patients seeking to avoid the harm that dentistry can do to health. Most of our callers are seeking to recover from the harm that dental mercury fillings have done. DAMS is a non-profit organization and does not endorse specific products or practitioners, but we do provide lists of dental professionals who subscribe to our way of thinking. They are DAMS professional members. Dr. Douglas Cook, D.D.S., of Wisconsin, is one such professional member of DAMS. He is among the best known and most popular biological dentists in the Midwest, and his patients come to him from far and wide.

Over a decade ago, I first began to hear of Dr. Cook because numerous patients in my state, Minnesota, had gone to him for safe amalgam removal and for the safe, carefully chosen dental materials that he would use to replace the mercury fillings. Later, I learned the key to his success: his use of computerized electro-dermal screening (CEDS) to probe the patient's body, to discover what the dental problems are, and where they are, and to choose the most compatible replacement materials. In this book, Dr. Cook seeks to share the secrets of his success – CEDS, low-speed drilling, and more – with any dentist who wants to learn them. I welcome this book, as I welcome the use of electro-dermal screening in dentistry. For all too many patients, including the sickest ones, such as those suffering from chronic fatigue syndrome and several chemical sensitivities, the usual blood serum tests for bio-compatibility are simply not valid. The CEDS method, used by Dr. Cook, has in my opinion, much more validity. I hope that the methods and the insights of Dr. Cook become widespread. The interested layperson will also benefit from this book and find it very informative.

Leo Cashman, Executive Director
DAMS
(Dental Amalgam Mercury Solutions)

Disclaimer

This book is educational, and is not to be used as a basis for medical or dental diagnosis and treatment. Douglas L. Cook, D.D.S., has based the information contained in the content of these chapters on experience and results with his patients, and review of the scientific literature. Dr. Cook's book is not intended to substitute for medical care by licensed health professionals. Treatment of individual health problems that may involve the oral cavity must be closely supervised by a physician and/or dentist. Dr. Cook does not recommend changing any current medications, altering any current therapies, or adding any new therapies without first consulting a qualified physician and/or dentist.

Chapter 1

New Solutions for Dentistry

In 1968, I changed to a metal free practice because of my dental assistant. One day my assistant said, "I love working here, but something is happening to me, and I don't know what, I have to quit working. I am so shaky; I cannot even write my name." Three years later after reading the story "Quicksilver and Slow Death", in the October 1972 issue of National Geographic, I immediately realized why my assistant had the shakes and why she had to quit working for me. The answer was mercury poisoning.

Mercury is a neurotoxin! Neurotoxins affect the muscles throughout the nervous system. Mad Hatters Disease was a common term used over a century ago to describe the affliction of the English hat makers who would dip their felt hats in mercury, allowing them to shape the hats with their hands. This procedure would cause the hat workers to lose control of muscle movements and they would throw their arms and legs around as though they were mad. My assistant was not that extreme, thank goodness, yet she knew something was wrong.

The "Quicksilver and Slow Death" article made me realize she was absorbing mercury though her skin while making mercury amalgam forms for crowns. She had been using her fingers to smooth the mercury amalgam dies from impressions of patient's teeth, thus sending the toxic mercury throughout her body and disrupting her muscle control.

It is said that when you are ready to learn, a teacher will appear. Throughout my dental career this has happened to me more than once. Because of the story, "Quicksilver and Slow Death", I began taking seminars that illustrated the relationship of dental materials to health. My wake-up call was learning the toxic effects of mercury in silver amalgam fillings. I soon began helping my patients become healthier by using non-metal fillings.

Another earth-shattering wake-up call happened when a patient brought an x-ray to me, showing an abscess on a root of a tooth supporting a bridge I had placed one year prior to this visit. I knew the filling was not that deep, and that the decay was not deep. Also, had I drilled into the nerve, I would have told her. I explained to her that *something* had caused the tooth to die, and that when I found the cause I would tell her.

Three months later, in September 1987, I witnessed the damaging effects of high- speed drilling when I attended a seminar in Carmel, California, headed by Dr. Ed Arana, DDS, head of The American Academy of Biological Dentistry. Dr. Ralph Turk and Dr. Fritz Krammer together gave a week long dental seminar. Halfway through the week Dr. Turk put slides on the screen showing the deadly effects of high speed drilling on the nerve of a tooth.

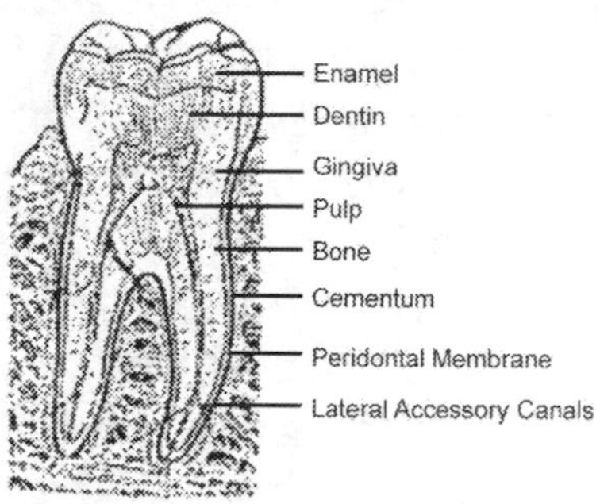

1.
Normal healthy tooth
Note: Auxiliary nerves

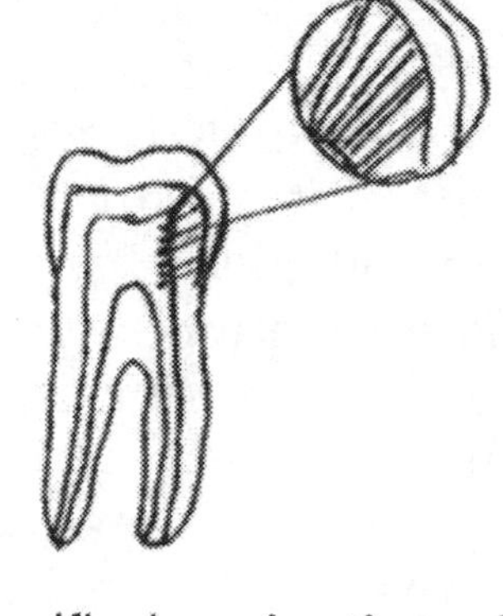

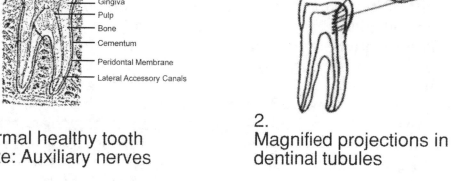

2.
Magnified projections in dentinal tubules

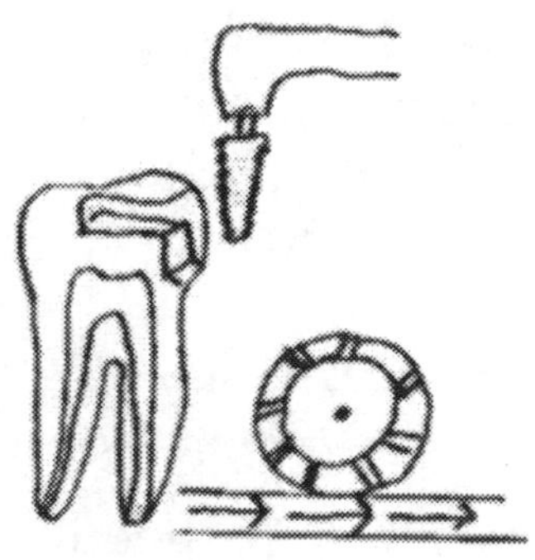

3.
Vacuum created from high-speed drilling, through the pulp canal

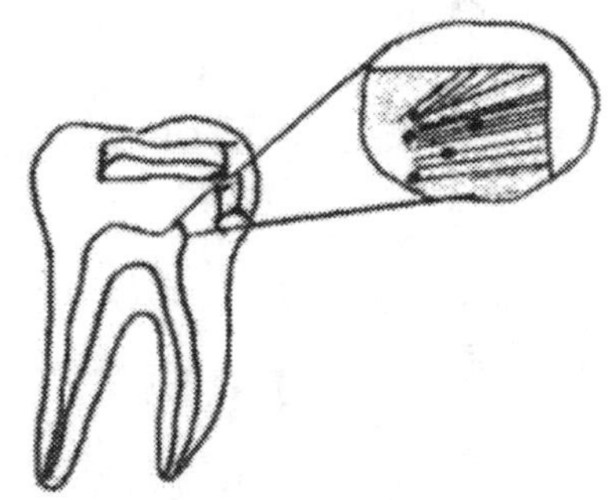

4.
Odontoblasts pulled out of dentinal tubules by high-speed drilling

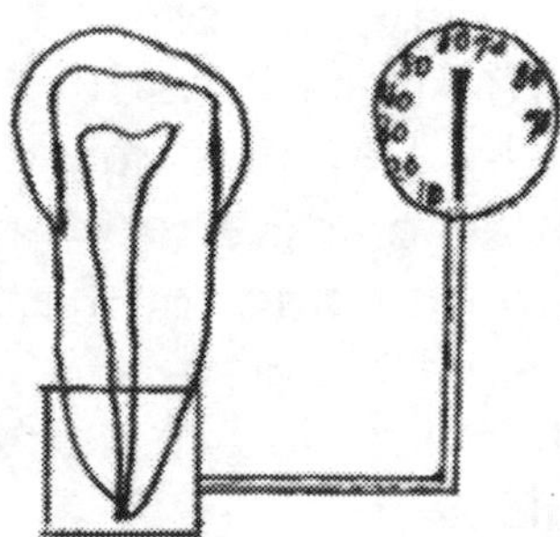

5.
Vacuum system to measure suction on odontoblast by high-speed drilling

Conventional dental hand-pieces (high speed drills) run at 350,000 revolutions per minute creating a vacuum that pulls the odontoblasts out of the dentinal tubules (picture 3 and 4 above). Consider that dentinal tubules extend from under the enamel into the soft pulp chamber inside the tooth (picture 2). This is a serious problem because, without odontoblasts the tooth is unable to repair or create dentinal matter. In a healthy, undamaged tooth, a tubule carries nutrients from the pulp chamber in the center of the tooth, into the dentine of the tooth. In a damaged dentinal tubule, bacteria can invade the tooth, moving in the "wrong" direction, passing through the dentine and into the pulp chamber. Bacteria can then pass through these tubules directly into the nerve chamber of the tooth causing an abscess (infection) which will likely kill the tooth. Picture 5, a diagrammatic drawing of a vacuum system used at Seamen's Lab in Germany, demonstrates how use of the correct drill speed on the tooth reduces sensitivity and helps save teeth.

<u>HIGH SPEED DRILLING was my answer to my patient's question for the loss of her tooth</u>.

I learned this information too late to prevent high speed drilling from killing ten of my teeth. In 1987, I removed my high- speed drilling equipment from my office forever! 20,000 revolutions per minute has been my top speed for the past thirty years, making patients more comfortable and saving teeth that could have been lost due to high speed drilling. And, yes it does take longer to prepare a tooth for a crown, inlay, or composite restoration; however, I have reduced the number of teeth lost by my patients. It is a fact that every dentist can save more teeth by using low speed drilling. I would rather take more time with low-speed drilling and save teeth, than lose one tooth to save time with high-speed drilling. Patients with dying teeth from high-speed drilling are sent to endodontists and general dentists to perform unnecessary root canals.

Millions of root canals are done every day in the United States adding to our nation's health crisis. This quote from Dr. Boyd Haley, at the University of Kentucky, Professor of Chemistry, and

Toxicologist (an expert at measuring toxicity), sums it up, "all root canals are infected."

To learn more on root canals and their effect, read *The Root Canal Cover Up Exposed!* by George Meinig, D.D.S., Bion Press ISBN 0-945196-14-8

Information on root canals can be found on the Price Pottenger Foundation website www.price-pottenger.org. Look for Weston Price's work on root canals.

Visit www.iaomt.com to read more about root canals.

Dentists are finding better ways to solve the unanswered questions regarding systemic problems that come from the oral cavity. Dentistry can make a difference.

Root canals, infected teeth, and dead teeth many times do not show up on an x-ray and may not produce clinical oral symptoms. Yet, if present, they do play an important role in causing health problems.

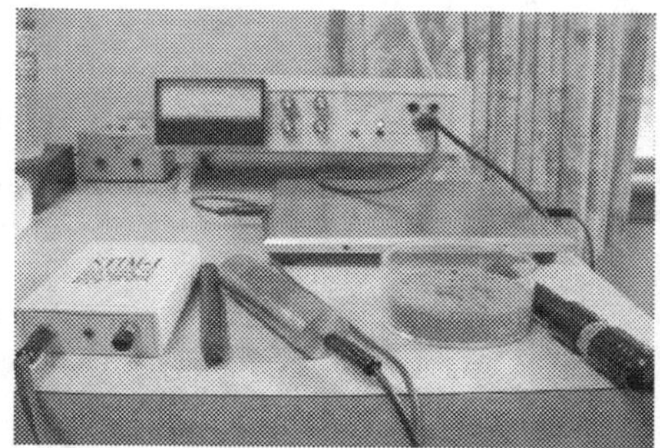

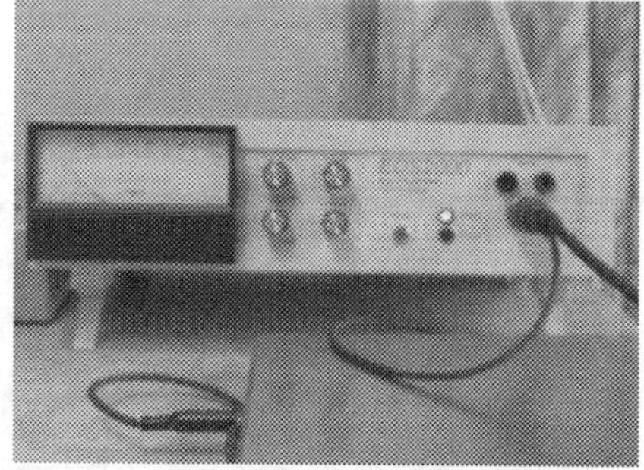

Photos of the Electro-Dermal Test System (EDS 2000)

Today, Computerized Electro-Dermal Screening (CEDS) is the most valuable instrument for finding sub-clinical dental problems. It is known as a bio-feedback instrument with multiple functions. Its major function is finding infection in the jaws (cavitations) and locating dead teeth. Using this CEDS instrument not only saves time and expense for patients, but is also an important key to good health. CEDS is also a valuable instrument to have in the office for finding energetically (energy) compatible dental restorative materials. Another important feature of CEDS is to check teeth for vitality (life) after all the metal, metal oxide fillings, and metal based crowns have been removed.

Balanced readings of fifty, on a scale of 0 to 100 indicate a good tooth and a healthy jaw area. A high reading of over 50 with an indicator drop will tell the patient and dentist that the jaw or the tooth is infected or showing signs of dying. All teeth are related to organ and tissue systems; it is a two-way street in which the organ can make the tooth painful or the tooth can cause the organ to look unhealthy. Observe the Teeth and Body Energy chart that correlates the teeth to bodily organs and systems. Many prescribing health professionals are not aware of these relationships. Patients may be given multiple prescriptions from medical doctors before the cause is found in the oral cavity. See the Teeth and Body Energy chart at the back this book.

Chapter 2

Teeth, Jaw, and Problems With Root Canal Treated Teeth

Health professionals and patients who understand the important relationship of teeth and jaws to body organs and tissue systems will see new solutions to health crises. Case histories are spread throughout these chapters describing the changes patients have experienced after having their fillings redone with compatible filling materials, and after removal of root canal treated teeth, jaw bone infections, and dead teeth.

Case: Aunt Mini, age 76, over-medication

Aunt Mini, after entering a nursing home, was soon unable to go to meals or the day room to play cards. Larry, her nephew, knew she had been in good health on entering the home. Larry had his doctor check her records, and found that she was on forty-one different prescriptions. Larry's doctor took her off forty of her medications, leaving her with just one. Two days later she was out of bed, walking to her meals and playing cards with all of her friends. Over-medication can result in the destruction of the immune system, poor digestion, gum problems and eventual loss of teeth. Refer to the back of the book for The Energetic Relations Of Teeth (Odontons) With Respect to Organs and Tissue Systems (Teeth and Body Energy Chart).

The oral cavity, for ideal health, must also be free of infected teeth and root canals. Pathology in the jaw bones, where teeth have been extracted or where the wisdom tooth should be does not always show up on x-ray, however the energy is still there and can cause poor health. Checking these areas with CEDS is essential for finding underlying pathology. Read more on this technique in later chapters.

Some of the problems associated with energy in the oral cavity are as follows:

1. All metal fillings and all composites that contain aluminum oxide, fluoride, and iron oxide can be a health burden. Barium in composites should also be checked with CEDS for compatibility.

2. Amalgam tattoos (black spots), are small particles of toxic mercury silver amalgam fillings that have been electrically drawn into the gum tissue.

3. Metal oxides in composites are an ongoing problem to all patients.

4. Tooth implants are not energetically acceptable in the oral cavity, and are the least acceptable way to replace missing teeth. Partial dentures and bridges are preferable to tooth implants.

5. In most cases pink denture acrylics contain toxic cadmium and may not be completely cured, potentially causing allergic reactions.

6. All metal partial dentures replacing missing teeth will lower body energy.

7. Any metal that crosses the midline of our body also affects energy. Example: jewelry, glasses frames, and metal partial dentures.

Problems 4, 5, 6, and 7 can affect denture patients who never feel well. The head and teeth are rich with acupuncture points and meridians (lines of energy, like electric wiring in a home).

After all other test results are normal, but the patient still says "I don't feel well", jaw and tooth evaluation may be necessary. Remember everything is energy resulting in various symptoms. Energy fields from fillings or temporaries can make both old and recent extraction sites look infected to the technician and health professional using CEDS. Follow my step-by-step protocol, to eliminate false readings. (Chapter 21)

Courses in CEDS are given by the American Association of Acupuncture and Bio-Energetic Medicine, 2512 Manoa Road, Honolulu, Hawaii, 96822 Tel. (808)-946-2069. Fax: 808-946-0378. Experience suggests that, if a dentist joins the Institutional Review Board (IRB), his/her licensing board will view the use of the CEDS instrument as legal and allowable for health research.

Case: Nanna, age 38, constant pains in the jaw and enlarged lymph glands in her neck.

Nanna's pain started after two infected lower first molar root canals (right and left) were extracted. Nanna developed a dry socket causing extreme pain, which was so intense that even strong pain medication did not relieve the discomfort. Nanna's physician could not find any bacterial problem that would cause her lymph glands to swell. Nanna called my office for an appointment for a CEDS evaluation hoping to find the cause.

Using the CEDS instrument, I found that both socket areas needed cleaning to remove residual infection. After this surgery, CEDS indicated improvement in both sockets. The next day, Nanna reported comfort on both sides of her lower jaw and her lymph glands had returned to normal. CEDS procedures are very helpful in understanding how filling materials and dead teeth can affect the total health of the body.

The most compatible composite dental filling material I have found for small fillings in a low stress area is Holistore. Because the filling material is not as hard as enamel, the patient's fillings need to be checked every six months to be resurfaced or replaced when wear is noticed. Holistore is made by Den-Mat. Holistore has no aluminum oxide, no iron oxide, no barium, and no fluoride. It is a highly compatible, metal free filling material.

Health is a major criterion for how missing teeth should be replaced. Important factors for success are the patient's home care with the necessary consistent cleaning habits and good nutrition. Tooth replacement can be done healthfully in one of two ways. We will describe each option.

Method number one: By bonding the bridge onto the abutment teeth (the ones holding up the weight of the bridge), we avoid crowning those abutment teeth. Crowning the abutment teeth causes a loss of enamel, thus weakening them and shortening their lifespan. Food collects around natural teeth requiring brushing, flossing, and flushing. Fixed or bonded bridges require the same care as natural teeth with the added need of cleaning under the false tooth held in place by the bridge.

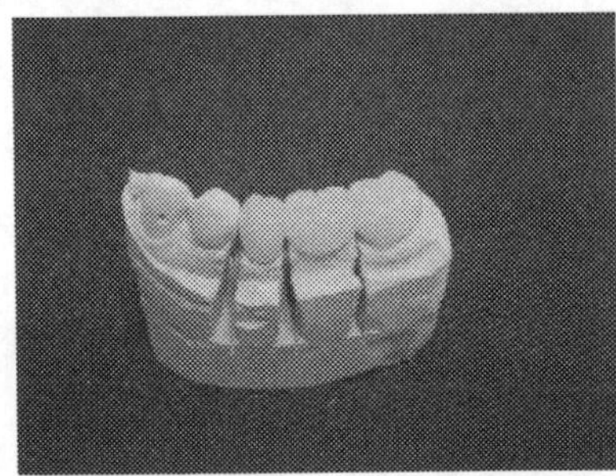

A Premise Indirect (formally BelleGlass) Bridge on the model and off the model.

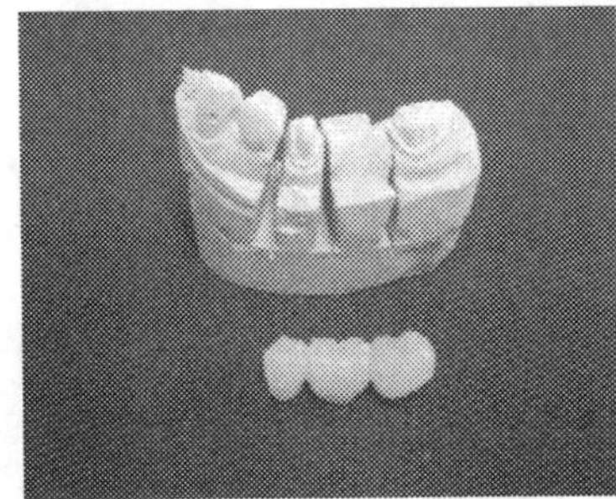

No metallic materials are used in this bridge.

Method number two: An upper and/or lower partial. First, an impression is made of the upper and/or lower remaining teeth and the impressions are sent to the lab, Cook Dental Lab (920-842-2083) where an all plastic partial is constructed to replace the missing teeth. These partials are made with cadmium free plastic. Cadmium is often used in partial or full dentures to give the plastic portion of them a pink tint, a gum-like color. But cadmium is a toxic material that should be avoided.

An important consideration for partials is how the natural teeth come together. Is there enough room for the partial, and are the remaining teeth healthy enough to hold one? With this information the dentist can make an intelligent decision to help the patient restore good chewing function.

An upper and lower partial and a bite splint made from cadmium free material.

A removable partial makes it easier to clean both the false teeth and your natural teeth after eating.

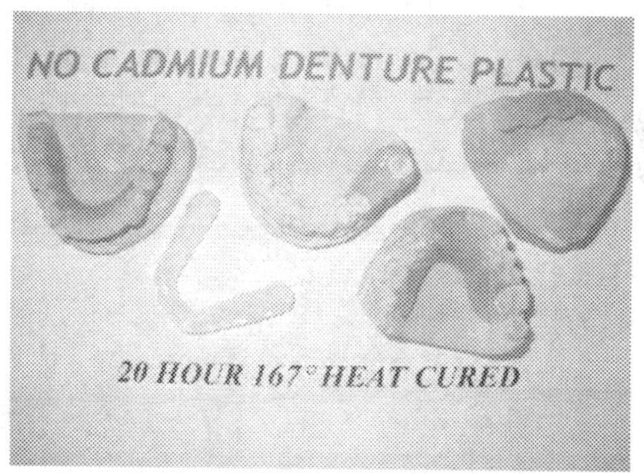

NO CADMIUM DENTURE PLASTIC
20 HOUR 167° HEAT CURED

Flossing your teeth requires being extremely fussy. Using a mirror six inches away from your mouth you will see the plaque being removed by the floss. **Floss only the teeth you want to keep!** Just before bedtime is the best time to brush, floss and flush (irrigate). See Appendix A in the back of the book for a list of water irrigating devices.

Dental materials used to restore or replace missing teeth need to be tested with CEDS for compatibility. Compatible dentistry may save patients from a lifetime of prescriptions and poor health.

For compatible partial and full denture material is cadmium free Vitalon 1060 and for restorations (crowns, inlays, onlays and bridges) unshaded Premise indirect. These Premise restorations can be shaded; however, the shading contains metal oxides. Only a few labs will make unshaded Premise indirect. Flint Cook Dental Lab is one of these labs that can meet your dental needs.

Flint Cook
Cook Dental Lab
10971 Clinic Road
Suring, WI 54174
(920)-842-2083

Partials need to be metal free, and cured in a hot water process for twenty hours at 167 degrees Fahrenheit. Other cured denture materials may be compatible; however all should be tested on the patient, using CEDS, prior to selecting one over another.

Three reasons why Dentures and Partials may be uncomfortable:

First, poor fit is a major reason most patients are not able to wear full or partial dentures. The supporting jaw bone must also be without undercuts, or sharp bone projections, as both will cause discomfort.

Second, the pink or clear material holding the teeth is not completely cured (cooked), or the material may not be compatible with the patient.

Third, plastics containing cadmium, a toxic heavy metal, may create a toxic energy field that can cause health problems in some patients. (Webber MM., 1985, Waalker MP Rehm Coogan

TP, et al, Cadmium in the human environment; Piscator M, 1981, Prostate cancer.)

A good fit and compatible denture material are necessary for the patient to be comfortable when eating a meal. A loose fitting denture can be caused by weight loss or a change in the fluid content of the patient's body. Menstrual cycles can cause some women to retain water. Taking an impression at the time of the greatest water retention, (i.e., a menstrual period or just before it) may cause the denture to feel loose after her period is over.

Case: Joan, age 33, a new denture.

Joan had a troubling experience after I made a denture for her. I took Joan's impressions just before her period, a time of her greatest water retention. Her entire body, including her gums, had changed in size. After four days, having lost this extra body fluid, she returned for the new denture. Her new upper denture, when placed, almost fell out of her mouth. I remade the denture when her period was over, and the fluids in her body had returned to normal. We were pleased with the end result. Her upper denture fit like a suction cup, for comfortable chewing, drinking and talking.

Information for the Dentist:

"Remember, *all* teeth are related to the first and second cervical vertebra and also to eye function." Dr. Reinhold Voll, M.D.

Read Carrie Smith's letter telling of her extreme dental experience.

> Dear Dr. Cook,
>
> I am finally writing to tell you the wonderful things that have happened since you finished my dental work last April. First, here is a big THANK YOU for doing such a

wonderful job. Besides my teeth looking beautiful, I am enjoying several health benefits. First of all, since you finished the work, I have had no more TMJ (jaw joint) pain! I can't say enough about that because the pain I used to get in my left ear was excruciating - like a sharp knife jabbing every few seconds to minutes. This would last anywhere from ten minutes to a couple of hours at a time. And sometimes this would be every day to every few days. It's so nice to be pain free.

Another bonus having to do with my TMJ is that I am no longer grinding my teeth when I sleep. This is big because I have been grinding for at least eighteen years according to the dentists and TMJ specialist I have been to over the years. I had a TMJ checkup with my dentist in Michigan (Gary DiStefano, an expert in TMJ disorders) twice since my dental work was finished - in May and again in October. I am happy to say that on both check-ups he said by looking at my night appliance I have not been grinding my teeth at all! The only thing I need to do for my TMJ now is wear my appliance at night. Thanks again for ending this pain and for saving me lots of money down the road. And I can only imagine the health benefits of not grinding my teeth every night. ☺

Another huge improvement from my new dental work is my digestive system getting on track. I used to have quite a bit of gurgling and gas in my abdomen and bouts of constipation. This has all subsided except for on rare occasions if I'm experiencing a virus or something out of the norm. It is nice to feel "normal" again after all these years of putting up with that.

Last but not least, I feel like I have more energy than I have had in years. I have made many improvements in my lifestyle and health routine over the past few years and I am convinced the dental work has helped a lot with my overall energy level and feeling of well being.

One last note about a root canal I had years ago. I had a root canal done on a tooth around sixteen years ago. Four years ago I had the root canal redone and it was still infected and painful. After researching and finding out how harmful root canals are I had it pulled. The day I had it pulled I remember walking out of the dentist's office and experiencing a clarity of vision like I hadn't before. I felt as though I was looking through a clear window where before it had been foggy. I thought maybe this was my imagination but day after day I had this new clear field of vision. As time wore on I became used to it but in the first few weeks after the tooth was pulled it was striking.

Another thing that was affected by pulling this root canal was that I have not had any more sinus infections (and I used to have them constantly on the side where the root canal tooth was). Needless to say I am very glad I had the tooth pulled and now have the beautiful bridge you put there.

I hope you are having some luck with finding a dentist to train in what you do. It is so needed! And so is the book you are working on. Please feel free to edit and use any of this letter for the book.

Happy Holidays to you and everyone in your office.

Sincerely,

Carrie Smith

Chapter 3

Oral Potential Meter II Reveals Hidden Health Problems

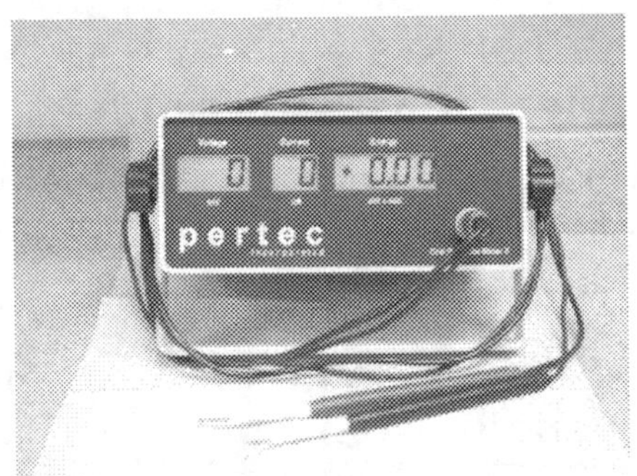

The Oral Potential Meter II

The Oral Potential Meter II is one of the most outstanding galvanic meters for health professionals today. Hidden galvanic electrical currents in fillings have far- reaching effects throughout our body. Many health problems are found with this meter that measures in electrical terms, (i.e. milli-volts (voltage), micro-amps (current), and in micro-watts times seconds (energy). Research is under way studying the relationship between electrical currents produced by metal fillings and pain. Other functions of the OPM are to indicate the presence of decay and ion release, as revealed by oral galvanism (electric current) in metallic restorations.

Health problems such as headaches, eye sight, fatigue, joint pain, foot pain, facial pain, mental fog, hearing radio signals, digestive disturbances, constipation, and diarrhea, can be caused by electric currents produced by metals in fillings, crowns and other dental metals.

Today's Dentist Can Help Health Problems

Today's dentists are taking their education and skills to another level. This new level relates to how dental services affect general health. Pick up any magazine, newspaper, or watch TV to find numerous articles on diet, drugs, and oral health risks. Notice the increased concern about the oral health of our population.

Patients are suspicious of prescription drugs and surgery, but rarely, if ever, do they have concerns about dental procedures and restorative materials. Though a trip to the dentist is considered safe, the oral cavity can be one of the major causes of sickness and various health problems. Remember Dr. Stone's opening statement at the beginning of the book. In recent years the public has become alarmed over the extensive adverse publicity regarding dental materials: root canal treated teeth, all metals fillings and metal oxides in composites.

Dental procedures such as root canals, implants, and the use of fluoride can be major causes of health problems. Recent studies point out conditions in the mouth may be linked to diabetes, strokes, pregnancy complications, circulatory and heart problems, and even to osteoporosis. As far back as 1754, Dr. Sulzer, a dentist, found galvanic (electrical) dental conditions in metal fillings to have far reaching effects on patient pain. Seventeenth and eighteenth century dentists were just touching the tip of the galvanic (electrical) iceberg.

I was deeply impressed with the Oral Galvanism phenomenon at an early age, when I experienced pain from a new mercury silver amalgam filling. Having my father as my dentist, I received all the very best mercury silver amalgams that a loving father could place to save his son's teeth. These same fillings today contain the same high content of mercury, 50% by volume of the mix, with the fine powder approximately 75% silver, and 24% tin, with small percentages of copper and zinc.

Multiple metals can produce an electrical condition resulting in pain. When biting my teeth together I experienced this electrical pain with my new filling. Eliminating this galvanic current and pain in my deciduous (baby) tooth required removal of the mercury silver amalgam and replacing it with a gold inlay. Immediately there was no more pain in my tooth. High galvanic current in teeth can cause the death of a tooth, another very good reason for avoiding metal fillings. Metals in the teeth can cause severe pain.

Case: Edward, age 38, painful upper molar.

Examination and x-ray pointed to a tooth filled with a large mercury silver amalgam. The Oral Potential Meter II registered a high charge of 256 milli-volts, 26 micro-amps, and 1.28 micro-watts times seconds. A normal reading is 10 milli-volts, 1 micro-amp, .01 micro-watts times seconds. Immediately, the electrical readings for the filling pointed to the major cause of Ed's extreme pain. Removal of the filling and placement of a compatible composite was completed without any complications. I explained to Edward that with the high current and extreme pain, it would take two or three days before the tooth would be comfortable. Ten years later the tooth is still healthy and Edward is still free of pain. He did not need the root canal or extraction that had been recommended by another dentist.

While attending the American Academy of Biological Dentistry seminar in 1987, I heard Dr. Krammer and Dr. Turk. They explained and demonstrated their version of a galvanic meter for displaying electrical currents in metallic fillings. Today's Oral Potential Meter II is more accurate and less expensive. Three large display windows display voltage, current, and energy, making it easy for both patient and health professional to assess the presence of electricity due to metal dental materials.

Dorland's Medical Dictionary cites the earliest discovery of electricity in fillings was made by a dentist, Dr. Sulzer in 1754. Dentists knew pain was a primary factor when mixed metals were placed in patient's teeth. Mixed metals in fillings often resulted in a sharp painful shock in the tooth, and caused the pulp to become inflamed and die. Early dentists also knew when only one metal filling material was used; it resulted in lower galvanic electrical current.

Using gold of the same content in all fillings is a good way to lower the battery effect causing of this electrical current in the teeth. A better answer is to use restorations that contain no metal or metal oxides, thus stopping painful electrical current. Dentists and other health professionals can check galvanic currents in metal fillings using the Oral Potential Meter II instrument.

Key features of the Oral Potential Meter II are:

- consistent reproducible reading,
- user friendly numbers display milli-volts, micro-amps, and micro watts times seconds (energy) of the electricity in the filling
- a battery source power supply
- measures ions of metal particles release per second from amalgam fillings, and locates decay.
- FDA approved for sale to health professionals

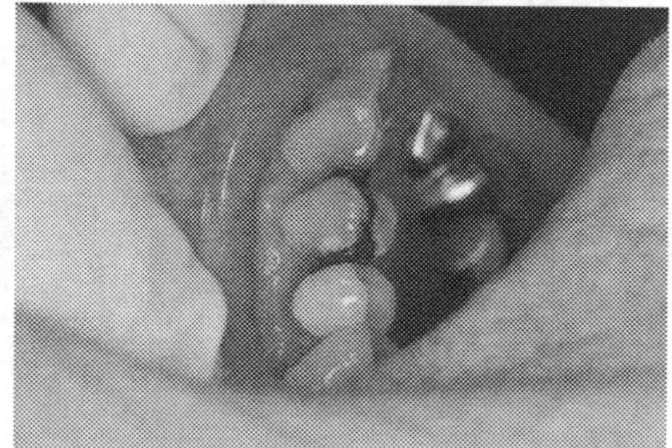

Dentists will notice margins of mercury silver amalgams are open on a surface that is easy to clean.

This happens because the electrical migration of the metallic ions, from mercury silver amalgam filling, carries with it calcium ions from the enamel leaving an open margin. This open margin will decay.

Note below: Plaque is sitting at the gingival margin (gum line) of the teeth. Plaque also has an electrical effect of pulling calcium ions from the enamel – resulting in decay. Plaque will eventually lead to decay.

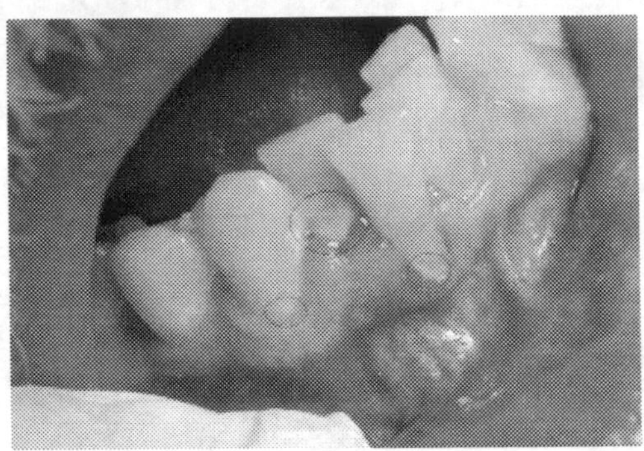

Subjective Symptoms of Oral Electricity

Every patient and health professional needs to be aware of symptoms that may come from electrical effect caused by metal dental materials such as: metallic or salty taste, increase in salivary secretion, burning or tingling sensation at margins of the tongue, nerve shocks and pulp sensitivity (made by a spoon or table fork touching a filling). Pathologic changes in the blood, kidney or other organs problems (caused by absorption of toxic metals) may be symptoms of galvanic current. Generalized discomfort in the mouth, irritability, indigestion, loss of weight and in some cases, reflex radiating neuralgic pains through branches of the fifth trigeminal nerve (in the head) may also be symptoms.

In the September 1936 volume of the Journal of the American Dental Association (JADA), Lain and Caugron wrote about that "galvanic pain", which is also known as an electro-galvanic phenomenon of the oral cavity, is caused by dissimilar metallic restorations.)

Dentists examining the oral cavity should look for the following signs of galvanic current: disintegration and discoloration of the metallic restorations, dental cement, redness with congestion and blanching of the mucous (soft tissue such as gums, roof of the mouth or cheek), evidence of intermittent or chronic irritation, sensitivity of the papillary bodies of the tongue, erosion area and ulcers on the margins, and denuded patches or geographic tongue. Leukoplakia is a grayish, slightly elevated pre-cancerous lesion, usually resulting from a long period of chronic irritation; this may be nature's warning before more serious pathologic processes develop. Even a small amount of current in the metal fillings can cause big problems. Go to the website www.metalpoison.net for more about the Oral Potential II meter.

Case histories have linked the battery effect from dental metals to the following symptoms:

- facial pain
- body pain
- loss of memory
- foggy brain problems
- digestive problems
- diarrhea
- depression
- hearing loss
- joint pain
- burning tongue
- bruxism
- grinding teeth day or night

Chapter 4

Harmful Effects of High-Speed Drilling

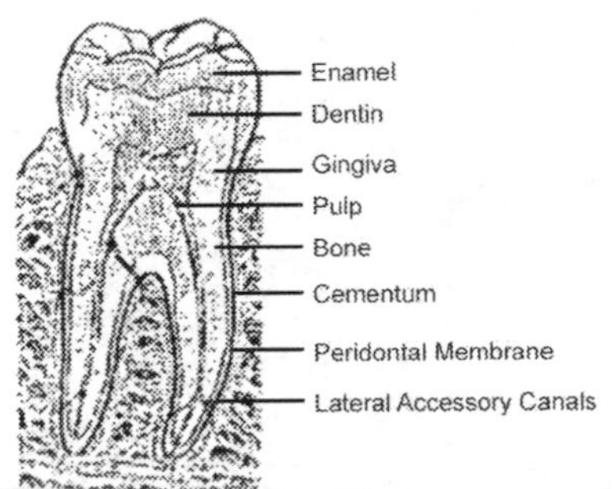

1.
Normal healthy tooth
Note: Auxiliary nerves

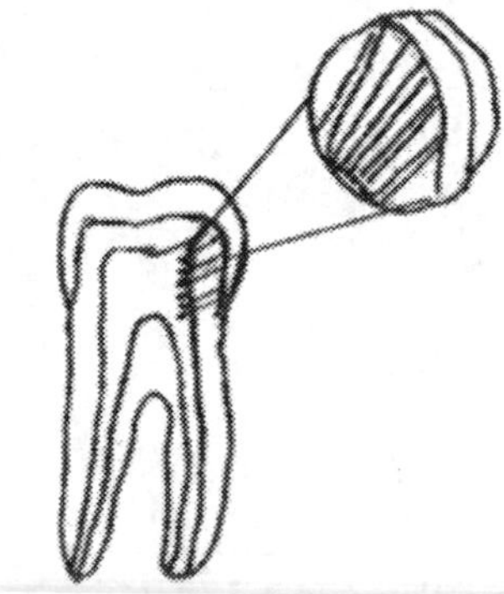

2.
Magnified projections in dentinal tubules

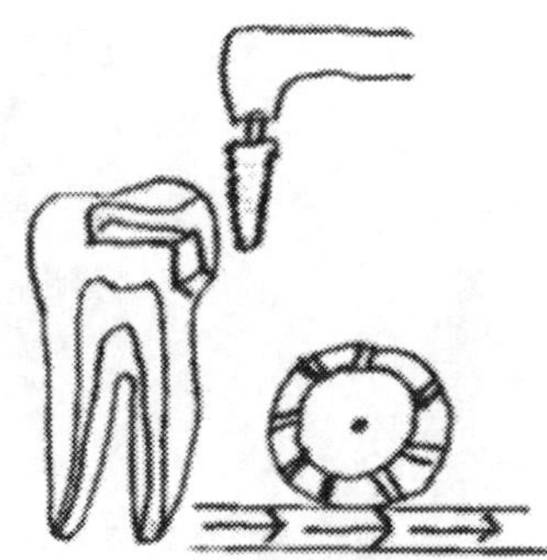

3.
Vacuum created from high-speed drilling, through the pulp canal

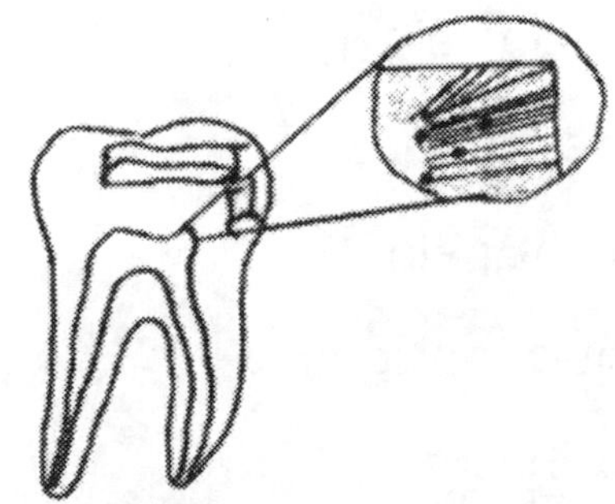

4.
Odontoblasts pulled out of dentinal tubules by high-speed drilling

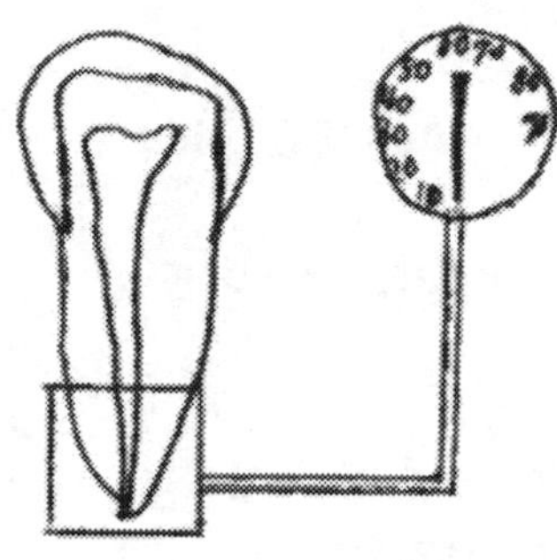

5.
Vacuum system to measure suction on odontoblast by high-speed drilling

Picture 1. A normal tooth, with its listed parts.

Picture 2. Magnification of projections in dentinal tubules under the enamel.

Picture 3. The drill creates a vacuum and heat when high speed drilling touches the surface of the tooth.

Picture 4. Odontoblasts (projections in the dentinal tubules) are sucked out by the high speed drilling.

Picture 5. A diagrammatic drawing of the vacuum test meter at Seamen's Lab in Germany. Low speed drilling creates no vacuum through the dentinal tubules.

High speed drilling results in a rise in temperature and creation of a pressure drop (partial vacuum) causes the loss of the tooth. Infection can start within a few days of high speed drilling leaving the dentinal tubules open for bacteria to pass into the pulp chamber causing infection. In my case, tooth loss did not develop a problem immediately. In some of the ten teeth I lost, the infection was present for three years before producing the clinical symptom of pain.

High Speed Drilling On Teeth,

Iatrogenic Effect (caused by dental procedures)

At a 1987 meeting in Carmel, CA, the American Academy of Biological Dentistry handed out this article:

Iatrogenic Damage Due to High-speed Drilling by Dr. Ralph Turk, D.D.S., Germany.

Reports by the World Health Organization (WHO) on the increase in chronic diseases are alarming! Dead teeth promote chronic disease.

According to the WHO these diseases have increased threefold over recent years alone. Environmental and civilization damage, such as stress, faulty diet, narcotics, alcohol, etc., also play a part in explaining the increase in chronic illness in the figures given by these statistics. Even if stress, stimulants and habit-forming luxuries have increased, this still does not sufficiently explain for the immense rise in the number of persons affected. Especially as cited both by the cheap press and more serious publications, many people are trying to keep fit through physical training and reasonable nourishment.

These personal health efforts on the one hand and the increasing consumption in stimulants plus the accompanying stress on the other hand, should, viewed statistically, balance each other out. If, in spite of this, such a horrendous increase in chronic diseases can be observed then WE, as physicians and dental specialists, are called to check why is this happening? Could professional operations also contribute to the fact that the number of chronically affected persons is increasing to such a devastating extent through the provocation of focal conditions? Every medical discipline has its inherent capacity to cause iatrogenic damage (doctor caused).

Dental work produces such a wide range of health problems that I am not able to report on all forms of iatrogenic damage. I would like you to think merely of the consequences of erroneous articulations reflected, or incorrectly performed, maxillary regulation, as well as badly fitted dentures or prostheses, fillings which are too high causing premature contact, fillings or pulp protection resulting in slow modification of the pulp, or mouth voltages produced by using different metals or alloys. All these forms of iatrogenic damage can result in severe negative effects on the general health of the patient.

I would like to encourage thought about forms of damage which have not been taken in sufficient consideration up to now, or those that might have been noticed, but have been deliberately ignored.

In the context of dental surgery, the primary and, indeed, principal consideration is the dental turbine or rotor. In my opinion and also, that of several university clinics, this should be considered as a sort of time bomb! Its devastating effects have been completely underestimated by most of our colleagues.

The (dental) industry has propagated the ergonomic advantages of these high-speed drills, constantly developing more functions; and without long-term clinical, histological or pathological monitoring of the effects of turbines in general, the entire dental profession, including universities, has adopted these diabolical machines.

How do turbines cause damage?

1. By the effects of grinding and drilling burs on the tooth enamel. The turbine does not grind down in the manner of slower machines, but rather breaks up the enamel prisms by impact, not only on the edges of cavities and preparations but also far down into the enamel that supposedly has remained intact: this has been proved by samples recorded through an electron microscope. The resulting cracks allow not only allow the spread of bacterial toxins but also the penetration of bacteria themselves and macromolecules into the dentine. This encourages caries. (ENCOURAGING CARIES)

2. But the major damage is caused in and on the dentine itself. Many colleagues are of the opinion that the pulp receives too much heat due to friction when turbines are used in treatment. Additional abundant cooling would avoid such a burden. A high rotation speed, causes both (a) congestion and low pressure vacuum occurs (on the dentine, a dry (or water-less) zone is formed at the very point of drilling or grinding/milling.

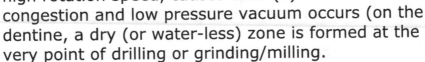

3. In an edition of a German-language journal (the ZWR), SCHOLER, a Swiss colleague described trials with air and water-cooler turbines: he discovered that, after 5-20 seconds of milling or grinding with turbines, an increase in pulp temperature by 12 degrees C (about 22 degrees F occurred, causing irreversible damage in 60% of the pulps examined. These findings have found their confirmation in an almost identical study by HENNING and PRZTAK, who are also mentioned in the same

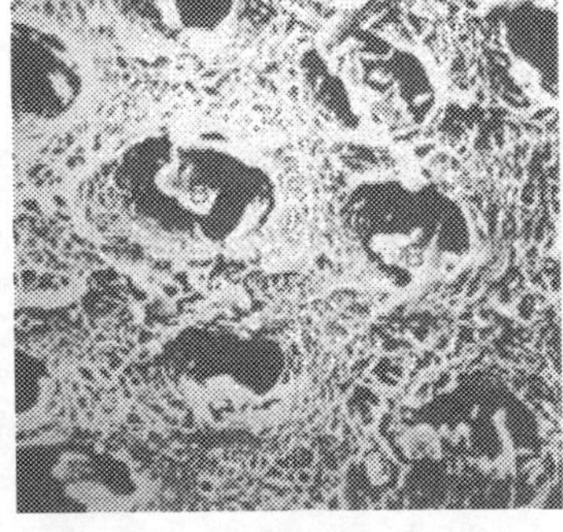

article. This article, however, did not mention another kind of damage, which is not produced thermally, but equally which spells doom to the pulp: damage from low vacuum pressure. (See above: Dentinal tubules under high power magnification, note B for bacteria).

As a result of the high rotation speed, turbulence is produced around the burs, which produces a very high negative pressure vacuum over the dentinal tubules (according to my own most recent tests this amounts to as much as a 10 mm water column per 100,000 revolutions). This negative pressure does not increase in straight-line proportion to rotational speed but rather exponential fashion: as a result of this state, the peritubular dentine linings, and the cylindrical odontoblastic processes are damaged and sometimes torn out, even odontoblast cores may even be partially sucked into the tubules.

Professor RAVNIK of Ljubljana in Yugoslavia was already able to prove this many years ago. This means that the metabolic processes in the enamel and dentine regions are disrupted decisively.

By way of reminder:

Approximately **5 million dentinal tubules** per square centimeter of cross section (equivalent to 12 million per square inch) are located in the crown area of the pulp. This number decreases down towards the root apex, although it still amounts to approximately 1.4 million at the cement limit. One single dentinal tubule has a diameter of 1.3 to 4.5 microns.

When the drilling or grinding bur is withdrawn, so that the negative pressure ceases, the empty and now open tubules can be filled in a retrograde manner by bacteria and grinding debris, as reported in English Language electron microscope studies. The denatured protein of the destroyed odontoblastic processes and cores can be broken down proteolytically by these bacteria.

If now, in the full light of this knowledge, we still consider how many colleagues apply their turbines day by day without hesitation on millions of patients. You are now able to understand why I used the phrase **"time bomb"!** By means of this machinery we are committing sin knowingly or unknowingly to a punishable degree against the health of our respective peoples!! At the present time, the results are unforeseeable. Is it not possible to say that a connection already exists between the turbine era and the precipitous rise in chronic illness?

For about 20 years now, turbines have been in use for grinding at least in 99% of all dental practices. It is a known fact that a chronic disease requires a longer time to develop. If one considers that pulp tissues die at a relatively slow rate and do not always immediately constitute a secondary source to the patient, they must, however, finally result in a breakdown of the local defense mechanism: this fact must at least be given some consideration.
In my opinion, the high-speed turbines, as presently used in dental practices, must be withdrawn from circulation at least in order to avoid damage of the kind described being inflated in the future. Our physical, physiological and histological examinations have shown that the upper rotary speed limit should be **20,000** rpm (revolutions per minute).

Bacterial toxins, capsular antigens and proteolytically broken down protein matter from the dental tubules act as antigens and result in permanent, auto-aggressive processes and finally in chronic irritation of the pulp. It thus becomes clear that the pulp tissues with damaged odontoblasts then have no chance of survival, and become the potential foci of problems of tomorrow.

In answer to assertions by colleagues to the effect that they only grind the enamel with their turbines, I would like to reply that they are in no position to determine macroscopically whether they are still working in the enamel or are already in the dentine. Even if the drill only contacts the dentine at one single point, the suction effect on the dentinal tubules then has already been produced, causing irreversible damage to the pulp. A partial statistic for ground or milled teeth speaks for itself: the application of conventional methods of pulp testing on teeth treated with turbines merely show changed sensitivity values, not whether the tooth is dying.

Measurement with CEDS is the only way to determine the damage in an exact manner. Responses to cold or heat stimuli, or to electric currents, (the usual clinical "vitality tests"), provide no evidence for the functionality of the pulp's vitality. I have been able to provide supporting evidence with test results involving histological examinations on extracted teeth, which had previously treated with turbines (high-speed drilling). High speed drilling is one of the main reasons teeth become sensitive to hot and cold, and can cause the teeth to die. A tooth that becomes sensitive after high-speed drilling can remain painful for days, or even months. Sensitive teeth should be watched carefully; if symptoms of discomfort increase, the tooth could be dying. CEDS should be used to cross check the sensitive teeth with their organ system.

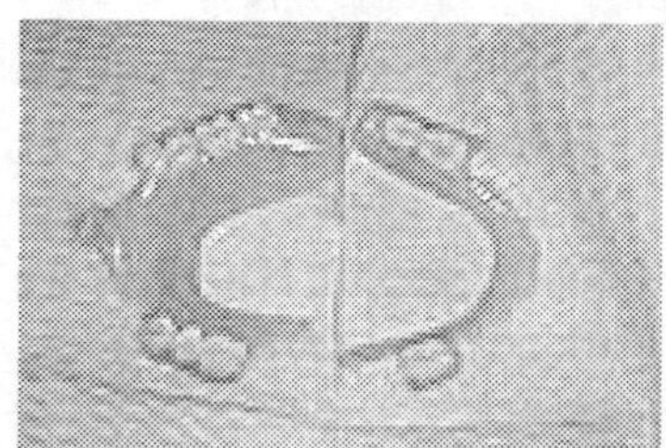

My teeth I have lost due to high-speed drilling and replaced with partials.

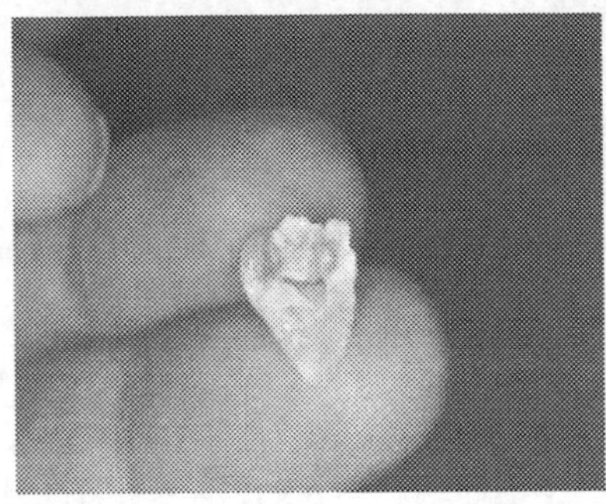

Infected Tooth due to high speed drilling

Low-speed drilling results in greater patient comfort after preparing the teeth for a filling, crown, inlay, or bridge. "Low-speed drilling" should be kept at 20,000 rpm or less.

Safe Amalgam Removal

Protection is needed while mercury silver amalgams are being replaced. Drilling out mercury silver amalgams creates toxic mercury fumes. Dentists can use two vacuum systems to remove nearly one hundred percent of these fumes.

1) One vacuum system, called Clean-Up (available from IAOMT), is used removing mercury amalgam fillings in the mouth placed over the tooth during the removal of mercury amalgam fillings to capture the grindings and fumes.

2) A second vacuum system held at the chin creates a vacuum over the face, pulling any remaining mercury fumes away from the dentist, assistant and patient.

Many dentists believe the rubber dam should be placed over the tooth while removing mercury fillings. Tests have shown that mercury fumes from the mercury amalgam pass through the rubber dam, as well as through the dentist's and assistant's rubber gloves.

Refer to Sherry Rogers's books, *Detoxify or Die* and *The High Blood Pressure Hoax* for what to take prior to having mercury silver amalgams removed. She also mentions a number of ways to remove heavy metals from the body. Safe, natural detox has to do with bowel transit of twenty hours or less. This is the time it takes for food to travel through and out of the intestinal tract after you have eaten. A longer transit time results in the recirculation of toxins and heavy metals, poisoning the body. Contact DAMS for the latest and most inexpensive ways to improve intestinal tract health and raise energy levels.

Removal of Metal Fillings

Most patients note changes after removal of mercury silver fillings, gold fillings, and base metal restorations (containing nickel), and replacement with non-metal or metal oxide free composite fillings. Some changes are: improvement in the immune system, gain in energy, sight improvement, vertigo corrected, heart symptoms improved, headaches gone with no need for medication, double vision back to normal, the clearing of mental confusion and anxiety, migraine headaches gone, nausea and chest pain gone, rapid and skipping heartbeat gone, back pain reduced, (with less medication or no medication needed), muscle pain in back and legs gone, sore throat from wisdom teeth gone, blood pressure returned to normal, and irritability gone.

Case: Sally, age 29, dry vomiting, itch on palate.

Sally's unusual case history resulted from a mercury silver amalgam tattoo (black spot on the gum) near tooth # 14. Amalgam tattoos occur when mercury ions, from mercury silver amalgam fillings, react with hydrogen sulfide (from infected gums) to form mercury sulfide, a black solid that is deposited in the gum tissue.

Sally had an itching sensation in the # 14 (1st molar) area and dry vomiting every day for two years, to the point of passing out. The 1st molar was a root canal with a mercury filling that had been extracted. Removal of the tattoo on the upper left side of the palate, next to where the 1st molar had been, stopped the vomiting and the itching sensation. Energy from the mercury tattoo and the relationship of the first molar to the stomach caused the dry vomiting. When she returned for suture removal she told me how pleased she was with the results. The itching sensation was gone and the dry vomiting had ceased.

Mercury Is a Toxic Element

Mercury, the second most toxic element in the world after plutonium, makes up 50% by volume, of the most common filling material, known as amalgam. An amalgam is, by definition, mixing mercury with other metals; but many people do not realize that fact.

When a Green Bay, Wisconsin high school had a mercury spill, the EPA (Environmental Protection Agency) was called out to clean up the hazardous material. Yet patients, uninformed about the toxic effect of dental mercury, allow this metal to be placed in their teeth. Solid scientific evidence has proven the harmful effects of mercury silver amalgams. Dentists and the public must demand a change to healthy restorative dental fillings.

Dentistry and Medicine

Dentistry and medicine can be brought together for the good of the patients. Few, if any, dental or medical schools teach dentistry from a health point of view. Along with all the established studies, one of the most important needs for the student is to understand the toxic effects of dental materials. Other health problems caused by root canal treated teeth, compromised teeth, and hidden infections in the jaws are not taught. Learning about these risks would help dentists and physicians protect their own health, as well as that of their employees and patients.

Fumes Come Off Mercury Silver Amalgam Fillings in the Mouth

At an International Academy of Oral Medicine and Toxicology (IAOMT) seminar, Dr. Roger Eichman, D.D.S. demonstrated how mercury fumes are given off by mercury silver amalgam fillings. Fumes immediately became visible on a fluorescent screen when Dr. Eichman scraped a mercury silver filling in front of a black light. All 200 attendees gasped in unison at the evidence of mercury fumes leaving the filling, like smoke leaving a lit cigarette.

Dr. Eichman explained that much more mercury vapor is released when patients chew, or brush teeth that contain mercury fillings. Published scientific papers report that the brushing of teeth and chewing of food typically increase the measured mercury vapor levels in the mouth tenfold. (Vimy, M.J., Lorscheider, F.L., 1985, Intraoral air mercury released from dental amalgam. J Dent Res 64:1069-1071)

Next, he demonstrated how mercury fumes arise from a gold crown by heating the gold. Gold produced the same methyl mercury fumes, and made a shadow of smoke across the fluorescent screen. Gold attracts mercury that migrates from the mercury silver filling! Gold crowns and fillings are easily contaminated by mercury and the mercury toxic patient who has gold crowns or inlays will not become mercury free until all the contaminated gold is also removed.

These same mercury fumes are emitted when new mercury fillings are being placed, or when an old amalgam filling is being removed. Knowing that mercury fumes are toxic, protecting the patient and the dental staff must be the dental team's primary concern.

To order "Smoking Teeth = Poison Gas", an eight minute DVD, call DAMS at 800-311-6265. This DVD clearly shows the mercury vapor coming off a mercury silver amalgam filling.

Dentists Must Know the Effects of Dental Materials

By understanding dental materials and the effects of these materials on a patient's health, dentists can make a difference. Mercury fumes can also cause various serious health problems for dental assistants and hygienists. Hygienists need the same vacuum system as dentists.

An Inexpensive Vacuum System

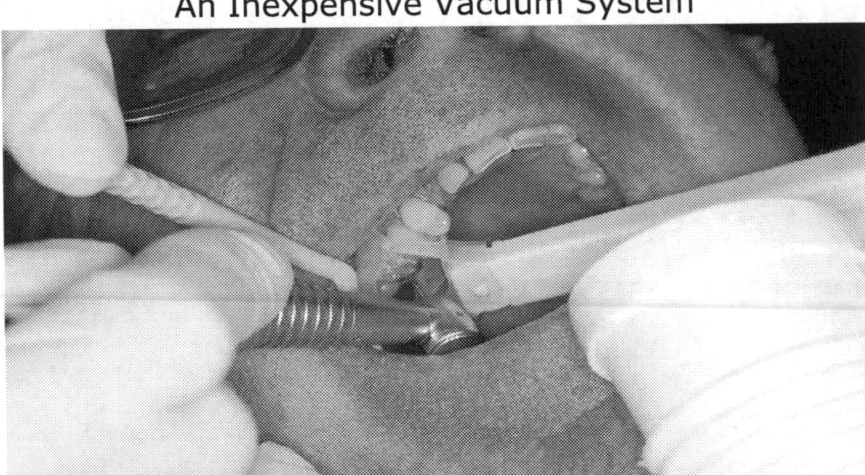

An inexpensive vacuum system can be made to pull mercury fumes away from the dental team. The cost of such a vacuum system is about $200.00, and may be purchased at any hardware store. Purchase a shop vacuum with both an intake and an exhaust opening. Place a pool hose on both intake and exhaust openings. One end of the hose will go to the patient and the other will be vented outside of the office. A vitamin bottle cap can be fitted to the hose going to the patient; three 1/4 inch holes are drilled in this cap allowing a negative airflow vacuum pull the air away from the patient's mouth and face. Suction removes the mercury vapor and fine amalgam particles from the mouth as the amalgam fillings are being drilled out.

The next most important step in removing the mercury amalgam and fumes is by using the Clean Up Tip, a plastic fitted barrier that surrounds the outside of the tooth. A strong vacuum attached to the side of the Clean Up removes the amalgam dust and mercury vapor. The high vacuum system that covers the tooth and is at the chin pulls the mercury vapor directly away from the patient's nose and mouth so the patient does not breathe it in.

One important fact about the use of a rubber dam: using an EPA approved Jerome mercury detector, it has been determined that mercury vapor passes through the rubber dam.

Chapter 5

Dental Office Location - A Practice Management Concern

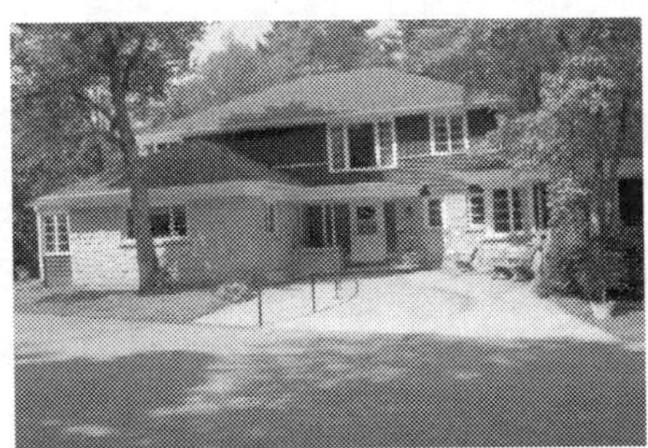
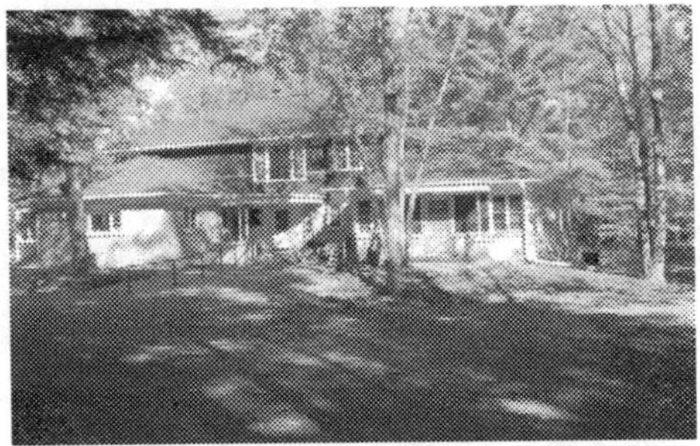
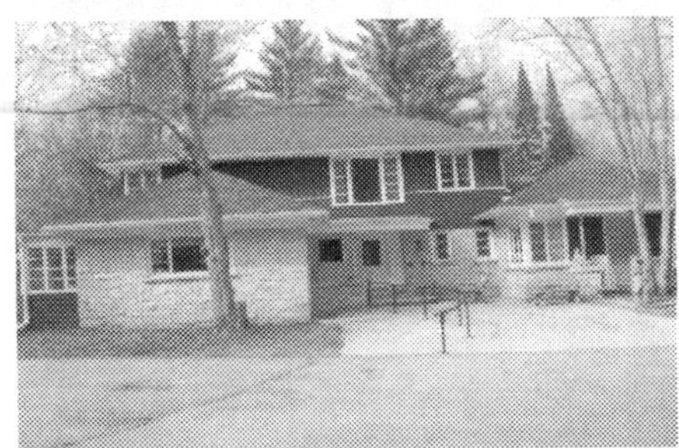
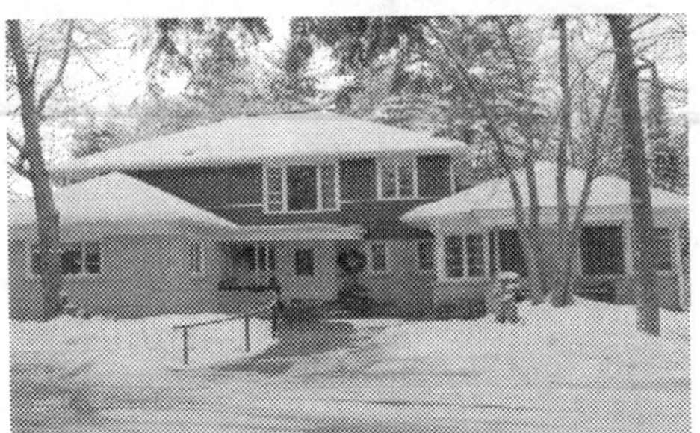

My office during the four seasons

Every course I have taken in practice management looks at the bottom line, "how much money can the dentist make?" I say, "how much good can the dentist do today, or who can they help?" Money will follow when you help those in need of good health through dentistry.

My father's dental office, on a trout stream near Breed, Wisconsin, became my office location. His dream as a young boy was a fishing shack on this very location; little did he know how his dream would come true.

He entered dental school after World War I, using money from the GI Bill to finance his education. He graduated in 1921 and started his practice in Gillett, Wisconsin. When the city of Gillett became crowded with a population of 1400, he decided to move north to his "trout stream dream."

After I returned from serving as an Air Force dentist in Germany, I started my general practice. My father's experience in oral surgery and dentures put me five to ten years ahead of most young dentists at that time. Continuing education added to my dental skills and knowledge. Fifty-five years later I am writing this book hoping to help patients and health care professionals fill a need by showing the connection between health problems and the oral cavity (odontons). Dentistry can make a difference.

Located in the woods, on a trout stream, my office allows patients and nature's wild animals to share this natural environment. Patients can expect to see deer, wild turkey, ducks, beaver, squirrels, partridge, and an occasional bear. For the trout fishing person, this place is heaven for fly or spin fishing. I find the stream relaxing in this fishing paradise. If I'm lucky, I catch a trout for the evening meal. This is a great place to help patients and to enjoy dentistry at a leisurely pace. I am looking for a dentist to join me in continuing this practice of dentistry and health.

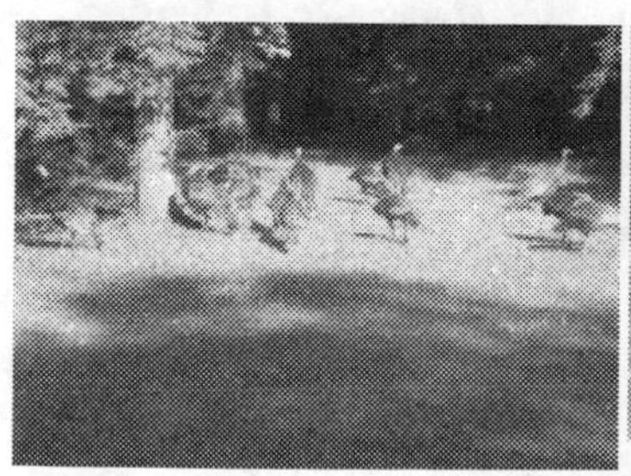

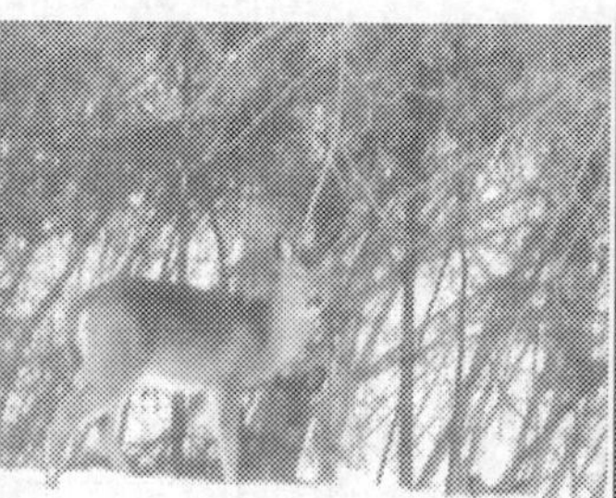

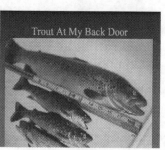

Little Was Known About the Dangers of Mercury Seventy Years Ago

Because my father was a dentist, I received 37 mercury amalgam fillings. Yes, I know there are only 32 teeth if you have all your wisdom teeth, but each tooth behind the six front teeth had one or more fillings. Sixty-five years ago my father did not know the dangers of mercury, and allowed me to play with it. He paid me to scrub his dental office, where droplets of mercury were on the floor from making silver amalgam fillings. The only thing that saved me from mercury poisoning was the scrubbing water that kept the mercury fumes from coming up in my face.

I learned in recent years of how mercury fumes came off my fillings and caused my immune system to become depressed. I had memory and vision problems, digestive and intestinal disturbances, all associated with mercury. It is common knowledge that if your immune system is weak, bacteria and viruses can attack your health at any time. Colds and sinus trouble were my main health problems. Food allergies also contributed to these problems. I was sensitive to dairy products and wheat gluten in grains. My parents, had they known, could have helped me with an "elimination diet."

During my four years in dental school, instructors had the same problem as my father in understanding the toxic effect of mercury fillings on students and patients. Dental school required the student to polish all mercury silver amalgam fillings in order to receive credit. One major toxic factor is that the heat and friction caused by polishing the fillings resulted in poisonous mercury vapor to leave the filling and to flow into the face of both patient and dental student. For more information, read the article "Quicksilver and Slow Death", National Geographic, October 1972.

In 1990, a CBS television show, Sixty Minutes, hosted by Morley Safer, delved into the amalgam mercury controversy.

Safer interviewed leading scientific researchers on the effects of dental mercury. He interviewed patients whose health had been significantly improved following safe amalgam replacement. He asked tough, probing questions of The American Dental Association (ADA) representative regarding their pro-amalgam stance.

Dr. Kristal's Immune Study with Dental Amalgams and Nickel Alloy

Dr. Harold Kristal, a California dentist, set out to prove that dental amalgams and nickel alloys reduce T-lymphocytes in the immune system. He used a thirty-patient study, taking a blood sample before and after the metal fillings was removed. Three months after removal, immune panels were taken, demonstrating each patient had an approximate doubling of their immune system.

The reason some patients and dentists are less affected by mercury comes down to two facts, one is fewer incidents of exposure, and the other is being able to detoxify mercury. A healthy diet aids in the removal of the heavy metals. In the book *Detoxify or Die*, by Sherry Rogers, M.D., the author explains how the use of anti-oxidants and chelating agents help to remove heavy metals from the system and restore good health.

Cleaning the intestinal tract, keeping the liver and kidneys healthy (Moritz 2005 fourth edition), using a far infrared sauna (Rogers, 2002), drinking good water to flush the acid radicals out (Batmanghelidj, 2006), along with exercise must be part of your health plan. All of our body cells demand good nutrition to support a healthy blood and lymphatic system, which help our body remain free of toxins. *Staying well is a full-time occupation.*

Chapter 6

Good Health Begins One Step At A Time

"Give your body half a chance and it will take care of itself."
I.L. Cook, D.D.S (my father).

I remember my father saying, "Give your body half a chance and it will take care of itself." His words pushed me to learn more than just the book-knowledge that Marquette School of Dentistry gave me. His deep interest in nutrition and health allowed me to see my patients in a whole different light.

When examining a new patient I ask myself, "If this were my mouth, with these health problems, what would I do for myself?" And the next question is "How am I going to help this patient become healthy with good dentistry and nutrition, and remove harmful heavy metals?"

My introduction to Computerized Electro-Dermal Screening started when a medical doctor suggested I attend Dr. Reinhold Voll's lecture in Atlantic City, New Jersey, in the fall of 1979. I left this seminar with the feeling that Dr. Voll's information could help a large number of patients. Dr. Voll's seminar encouraged me to go to thirty additional basic seminars, given by his student teachers in this country. Since then, I have continued to learn more about the oral cavity and its tremendous influence on the human body.

Dr. Voll stated that 80% to 90 % of systemic health problems are either caused by, or influenced by the oral cavity (teeth, tonsils and sinuses). His profound statement made my ears perk up. With these percentages the dentist is in the ideal profession to help his patients. After twenty-five years as a general dentist, and using the approved materials of the American Dental Association, I realized that these materials were causing serious patient health problems. I started looking for a healthy alternative to mercury silver fillings, knowing that most patients did not realize that the silver amalgam fillings in their teeth contain mercury.

Dentists do not see their patients when they become ill from restorative work. Restorative work includes mercury silver amalgams, gold foil (pure gold), gold restorations, base metal crowns (containing nickel, a known carcinogen), inlays, bridges, and implants as well as denture plastics containing cadmium. Many of the tooth-colored filling materials, called composites, contain aluminum oxide, iron oxide, fluoride and barium (a heavy metal and a radio opaque substance for x-rays); all of these can negatively impact good health.

All materials used to restore teeth affect the energy flow in our body. Because energy is produced by these filling materials, they must be chosen based on their compatibility with the energetic flow of the patient's body.

Chapter 7

Computerized Electro-Dermal Screening: What Patients and Dentists Need To Know

A major value of Computerized Electro-Dermal Screening is that it is a fast accurate way of evaluating the patient. CEDS aids the dentist in finding the most compatible dental materials, and in locating infection in teeth and jaws.

Dr. Voll discovered this bio-feedback system in 1954. His Electro-Dermal Screening instrument has gone through many changes since then. Today's instrument is responsible for gathering information in an easy-to-read form, similar to a blood pressure cuff. It does not diagnose; diagnosing and treatment is the responsibility of the health practitioner.

Health professionals must be registered under an IRB (Institutional Review Board) to legally use this instrument. To sign up for this, contact The American Association of Acupuncture and Bio-energetic Medicine Institutional Review Board (IRB): Phone 808-591-2345. A research program is set up to help health professionals determine the condition of the oral cavity. Research projects require a signed consent form from the patient and a recording of their readings. It is also important to keep a record for the IRB of any adverse patient reaction in connection with the CEDS

Appendix B at the back of this book contains The Energetic Relation of Teeth (odontons) With Respect to Organs and Tissue Systems Chart, or The Teeth and Body Energy Chart. This chart illustrates the relationship of teeth to the patient's organ and tissue systems.

One of Dr. Voll's favorite statements is, "If you know only one thing, know the Teeth and Body Energy chart." Know the two-way street, which is the relationship of organs to teeth and teeth to organs.

A good example of the relationship is the fact that the pain we feel in upper teeth often comes from a sinus infection. If we clear the infected sinus; the tooth pain often goes away. It is also true that an infected tooth will cause a painful sinus or joint pain; remove the tooth and the pain disappears. Stomach and joint pain can suggest that there may be infection in a related tooth. Infection in the jawbone associated with the stomach can also cause the same discomfort. A bad tooth can cause neck or back pain. Notice on the tooth chart that all teeth are related to the first and second cervical (neck) vertebrae. Dr. Stone had many patients tell him that their back pain left after removal of their metal fillings.

Case: Fred, age 48, stomach and joint pain.

Tooth # 29 an edentulous area, (the tooth was gone) is on the stomach conductance point of the lower jaw. Infection in jaw area # 29 was located with CEDS. Cavitational surgery and removal of infection stopped the stomach and joint pain. Knowing the association of teeth to organ and tissue systems (as seen in The Teeth and Body Energy chart) will help you see how pain problems anywhere in the body may be connected to the oral cavity.

Practitioners of Chinese medicine knew the importance of these "paired organs" and we as dentists must also know how liver and gallbladder, large intestine and lung, heart and small intestine, kidney and genito-urinary area, stomach, spleen and pancreas are connected, to understand how to help our patients.

The references listed below are for health professionals as well as patients who would like more information on the relationships between teeth and organs. Armed with this knowledge you can find answers to health problems that may otherwise go undetected.

Refer to *Interrelations of Odontons and Tonsils to Organs and Tissue Systems* by Dr. Voll ISBN 3-88136-064-6 www.redwingbooks.com

An Electrodermal Analysis of Biological Conductance by Vincent J. Speckhart, M.D. (H) ISBN 0-9741533-0-3 Biological Conductance Inc. 1340-1272 N. Great Neck Road, Box 188 Virginia Beach, VA 23454 U.S.A. (bioconductance@verizon.net)

As referenced on The Teeth and Body Energy Chart, the upper wisdom teeth are associated with the central nervous system, limbic system (mental attitude) and heart. Lower wisdom teeth are associated with the peripheral nervous system, kidney, small intestine, and heart. Dr. Voll said, "Wisdom teeth are related to heart problems 100% of the time." Infection in the jaw bone or a cavitation can be a result of a wisdom tooth extraction or where a wisdom tooth never appeared. The energetic effect (from infection) on the heart and associated organ and tissue systems can be a major problem. Wisdom teeth also have an energy effect on kidney, small intestine, ears (vertigo), mental attitude, and energy level.

Have your Teeth and Body Energy Chart nearby to follow each tooth and organ system: refer to upper right # 2 and # 3 molars, upper left # 14 and #15 molars - lower right, #28 and #29 bicuspid, lower left #20 and #21 bicuspid. The stomach and pancreas, each important to digestion, along with the spleen are associated with these eight teeth. Disturbed energy flow from fillings, root canals, dead teeth or cavitations in these locations can cause digestive problems.

Case: Lauri, age 38, radio sounds in her head

The oral cavity is the most overlooked area of the entire body when it comes to diagnosing illness. Lauri's hearing problem began when she walked into her bathroom and heard television and radio sounds. Lauri's problem is common when incompatible metal filings or oral infections are present. She had consulted many health practitioners about this undiagnosed condition, with no solution. The patient's doctor, Dr. Tom Stone, a physician knowledgeable about the oral cavity, referred Lauri to me for evaluation and treatment.

I recorded very high readings using an Oral Potential Meter II to measure the electrical currents in her mercury silver amalgam fillings. Our plan involved removal of the amalgam fillings that contained the high electrical current. After removal of the fillings she noticed that the radio and television sounds in her ears had gone away.

She sent me the following thank you note saying: "I had all but given up hope of ever finding anyone who could stop all the noise in my ears."

Sometime in 1987 I noticed a very distinct noise in my right ear. After a year or so the noise seemed to be gone, but I now realize that there was just a variation of the noise that I became accustomed to as background noise. In 1999 I began having an intermittent humming or buzzing sound in my right ear that went on constantly and became extremely annoying. Shortly thereafter I began having pain in the right side of my head and on the right side of my face and jaw. I also began having problems with my right eye. I had a constant indescribable sick feeling in the right side of my head. I had problems sleeping because of the noise in my ear and the pain in my head. I tried sleeping with either cotton or my finger in my ear at night to stop the noise. For the next several years I took aspirin every night before I went to bed and another dose in the middle of the night to stop the pain so I could get some sleep. I found myself constantly pulling the right side of my jaw apart. I would wake up at night pulling my jaw apart. The pain and problems with the right side of my head, face and ear had become unbearable.

I went to my ophthalmologist complaining of pain in my right eye, trouble keeping my eyelid closed at night and feeling that my right eye could not relax. He could find nothing wrong.

Every six months when I went in for my dental cleaning and check-up, I told my dentist about the pain in the right side of my head and face, the pulling on my jaw and the noise in my right ear. He had nothing to offer.

During the next 5 years I was shuffled from ENT's, to neurologists, to oral surgeons/dentists, to physical therapists. After getting no answers or relief from local practitioners, I sought help from the well known medical facilities. I was seen at Mayo Clinic, University of Iowa Hospitals, Barnes Hospital in St. Louis and the University of Chicago Hospitals. I saw a total of six oral surgeons/dentists or dentists specializing in facial pain, five neurologists and six ENT's. All types of tests were performed including a CT scan of my head and sinus, MRIs of my brain, trigeminal nerve and tempromandibular joints, MRI angiogram of my head and neck, EMG's, carotid artery ultrasound, hearing tests and blood tests. When all the test results came back normal, I was referred to another specialty or I was given a prescription for an anti-depressant, muscle relaxant or pain medication. None of these helped and some even made me worse. No one could offer any explanation as to what might be causing my symptoms.

In September 2003 I was referred to an oral surgeon who after ordering several months of physical therapy for myofascial release with no results, thought that all of the different metals in my mouth could be causing a problem. The possibility of the metals in my mouth causing my symptoms led me to Dr. Cook.

I saw Dr. Cook in August 2005. Dr. Cook measured the levels of galvanic action in my teeth. A gold crown on tooth #2 had a very high reading. When he removed this crown an amalgam filling which had been left in the tooth came out with the crown. I felt immediate relief in the right side of my head. All of the noise in my ear stopped. The pain and sick feeling in the right side of my head is gone. The constant urge to pull apart the right side of my jaw is gone. The pain and problems with my right eye have stopped. I am finally able to sleep at night without all the pain and commotion going on in the right side of my head.

After being told everything from I would be on prescription medication possibly for years, to I needed a neuropsychologic evaluation, to being told nothing at all; I cannot thank Dr. Cook enough for the relief he has given me.

I give Dr. Douglas Cook permission to use my story and my treatment.

August 30, 2005

Lauri K. Barton

Lauri K. Barton

Lauri's case is a good example of solving a hidden problem by being able to measure the electrical current in metal fillings with the Oral Potential Meter II.

Electrical current from fillings and infected teeth played a crucial role in Dorothyann's body pain.

Case: Dorothyann, age 59, pain in the sternum, stomach and sinus

Dorothyann came to me in 2006 with the above pain symptoms. We tested her on the CEDS unit to see if she had imbalances related to the oral cavity. I ended up extracting eight dead teeth and replacing her metal fillings. After all the work was completed we re-tested and found a cavitation in the # 1 wisdom tooth area. After we did the cavitation surgery all of her symptoms were gone.

She noticed her breathing was better, her sleeping was better, stomach was better, and her sternum pain and sinus problems were gone. Dorothyann sent me the following letter about her dental-related healing story.

Dr. Douglas Cook
10971 Clinic Road
Suring, WI 54174
June 29, 2007

Dear Dr. Cook,

I never dreamed that going to the dentist would be such a life- changing event and that my teeth are responsible for my overall health.

When I moved to Wisconsin 11 years ago from California, I had to search for alternative Medical help that was very prevalent where I came from. I had many aches and pains I thought were from my life as a professional figure skater. Plus, I seemed to have allergy attacks all the time. Not to mentions my lack of energy and state of "walking in a mental fog" most of the time.

I have a long history of dental work, since the age of 12. My mouth was filled with bridges, crowns and inlays that had all been replaced 3 times. I had braces for TMJ and the list goes on. I even flew back to Los Angeles to have a loose bridge repaired.

In 2005 I had an abscess under the anchor tooth of the bridge and was convinced to have a root canal on a previous root canal. Only now have I learned how very dangerous that was. I was very sick; major stomach problems from the antibiotics. I tried everything to heal because I do believe the body and spirit are powerful and capable of healing. I tried acupuncture, Chiropractors (which resulted in Cosotchondritis), Medical Doctor's who diagnosed Fibromyalgia as a possibility, vitamins and diets.

Thank goodness I heard about you through my acupuncturist and a dear friend who owned an Inn where your patient's from out of town often stayed. I know people come to you for dentistry from all over the country and the world. How fortunate you are 20 minutes from me.

I started feeling better with each extraction due to all the infections and removal of metals. The healing process was such a surprise, using natural herbs and nutrition instead of the antibiotics and pain medications that caused me so many problems.

I can't say enough about what you have done for me. Your passion and enthusiasm for your work is an inspiration and certainly proven by me. I have more to learn regarding nutrition and my total health but my pains have improved 100%. You are a great teacher.

I will miss coming to the Dentist on a regular basis. How many people can say that? Your office setting nestled in the woods, and your wonderful staff; Amy, Michelle and Melissa have made "going to the dentist" a most pleasant experience.

Thank you Dr. Cook,

Dorothyann Nelson

Effects of Filling Materials

Health professionals must know the effects of filling materials. But knowing the composition of the dental materials is only half of the story. The health professional must also know the energetic effects of these filling materials on the nervous system, immune system, mental functions, and digestion, and know how to eliminate heavy metals from their patients' bodies. Computerized Electro-Dermal Screening will aid in the search for compatible filling materials and in finding jaw and tooth infections.

Patients tolerate very few dental materials. Restorative filling materials do not affect all patients the same way. Example: metal gives off frequencies when you use a metal detector to find treasure at the beach. You might ask how the metal detector knows there is metal. The answer is ENERGY. Fillings in our teeth have energetic effects and the filling materials used must be compatible with each individual's energy system. Use of compatible filling materials is critically important to a patient's health.

Case: Ann, age 17, no cognitive functions

Ann, a beautiful 17-year-old girl did not know her right hand from her left. By the time her parents took her to a Dallas hospital her cognitive functions were basically gone. Tests were done and medications were given to try to help her regain her normal mental functions. This fruitless adventure ended up costing $70,000.00. The physician in charge of her case told her parents she would have to be put into an institution until they could figure out a treatment that would solve her problem. The mother suggested that they take her off all medication, and she would take her to another physician. Ann's mother took her to Dr. Thomas L. Stone, M.D., who was in the Chicago area at the time. With the use of the CEDS, Dr. Stone found Ann was being poisoned by aluminum. He used chelation therapy, by means of an intravenous drug to remove the aluminum from her body. With each treatment her mental functions improved.

Dr. Stone sent Ann to a Chicago dentist to have her mercury fillings removed and replaced with non-metal fillings. Following her dental appointment she relapsed to the same mental state as when she walked into Dr. Stone's office. With Dr.Stone's knowledge of dental fillings, he found the problem immediately: the local dentist had placed a composite that contained aluminum oxide, iron oxide and fluoride, materials that were very toxic to Ann.

Dr. Stone, knowing the cause of her problem, sent her to me to have compatible filling materials placed. Ann then returned to Dr. Stone's office to complete her aluminum detoxification, which allowed her to regain her mental functions.

Ann came to see me in 1993 for help. In 1996, Dr. Stone and I each received a letter from her telling us of her acceptance to Medical School. In the year 2000 she graduated with her medical degree. Her case emphatically points out the degree of sensitivity a patient can have and the need for CEDS.

Chapter 8

All Metals Carry Electric Current, No Metals Are Compatible

Do you have gold fillings? Dental gold is not pure gold; pure gold would be too soft for a filling. Gold must be durable enough to withstand chewing and support bridge work; therefore gold alloys (combinations of gold with more than one metal) are used to increase strength. As with silver amalgams, gold alloys can affect the nervous system. According to *Boericke's Materia Medica*, gold can cause depression and other physical and mental problems. Dental gold is an excellent restorative material with respect to durability, but is not the best choice of material from a health standpoint. Finding a compatible metal for fillings has proven to be impossible, if good health is to be a consideration. Metal fillings are a prime cause of a variety of health problems. In addition, not all patients will have the same health symptoms from the same dental filling material.

Case: Dr. Dave, D.D.S., age 55, migraines

Dr. Dave heard my presentation on dental materials at Dr. Simon Yu, M.D.'s seminar in St. Louis, Missouri. Dave arrived at my office, after a long nine-hour trip, with a splitting migraine headache. I put him to bed with an ice pack, hoping to give him some relief. After he had an hour of restless sleep I gave him an oral exam and a treatment plan. Using CEDS, we found all conductance points (acupuncture points) registered above fifty with an indicator drop. Our plan was to remove his gold inlays and crowns, leaving one pure gold foil in his front tooth. We started his dental work the next day and completed the removal of the gold inlays. Impressions were taken and un-shaded Premise Indirect (formally BelleGlass) restorations were finished in Flint Cook's Dental Lab. This Premise Indirect (BelleGlass) is 80% glass and 20% resin binder *without* an iron oxide shade. What is iron oxide? Iron oxide gives color to the filling material matching the patient's own tooth shade; iron is a heavy metal and iron oxide was incompatible with Dave.

Dave's headache improved, though it did not completely go away. Dave was checked again with CEDS to measure the energy effects of the pure gold foil filling; this was the last filling to be removed from his teeth. After removal of this gold foil (pure gold), a measurement with CEDS indicated why his headache had stopped. Two things were noted, (1) his headache had been reduced by 90 %, and (2) his high CEDS readings had returned to normal. Thirty days after his appointment I called David and found that he was comfortable and had a higher energy level.

Nickel Is a Toxic Metal

In 1984 Dr. David Eggleston, D.D.S., took blood samples to check the immune system of a patient who had nickel and mercury silver amalgams restorations. Following removal of the fillings and placement of composite fillings, another blood sample was taken and the patient's immune system function, as measured by T-cells, had nearly doubled.

Sterzl I, et al, Mercury and nickel allergy: risk factors in fatigue and auto-immunity, *Neruoendocrinology Letters* 20: 221-28, 1999.

Loken, A.C.; Lung cancer in Nickel workers. *Tidsskr NorLaegeferen* 70:376, 1950

Fursi, A., Haro, R.T., and Schlauder, M., Experimental chemotherapy of nickel induced fibro-sarcomas. *Oncology* 26:422, 1972

Gilman, J.P.W., Metal carcinogenesis II W study of the carcinogenic activity of cobalt, copper, iron, and nickel compounds. *Cancer Res* 22:158, 1962

Dr. Eggleston took this experiment one step further to prove his point that metals adversely affect the immune system. Mercury silver fillings were placed in the patient's composite fillings, not touching the tooth. Another immune panel was taken and Eggleston found her immune system had decreased by half. His findings are in the following published article:

Effect of dental amalgam and nickel alloys on T-lymphocytes: Preliminary report

David W. Eggleston, D.D.S.*
University of Southern California, School of Dentistry, Los Angeles, Calif.

The purpose of this research project was to determine the effect of dental amalgam and nickel alloys on human T-lymphocytes.

T-LYMPHOCYTES

Lymphocytes are white blood cells produced in lymphoid tissue throughout the body.[1] Some lymphocytes that pass through the thymus are activated or modified by the thymus and become T-lymphocytes.[2-4] Ideally, 70% to 80% of total lymphocytes are T-lymphocytes, but 53% to 80% is considered normal.[5]

Human T-lymphocytes can recognize specific antigens, execute effector functions, and regulate the type and intensity of virtually all cellular and humoral immune responses.[2-4, 6-8]

Two major functionally distinct subsets of T-lymphocytes have been demonstrated with heteroantisera, autoantibodies, and monoclonal antibodies directed at stable cell-surface antigens.[2, 3, 6, 7, 9-13]

The "helper" T-lymphocyte, also called the helper T-cell or T4-lymphocyte, is responsible for "labeling" or identifying cancer cells, pathogenic microorganisms, and foreign bodies. Macrophages and other white blood cells cannot combat these materials until they have been labeled by a T4-lymphocyte. Therefore, a malfunction or reduction in the number of T4-lymphocytes results in a depressed immune response to antigens.[2-4, 6, 7, 11] An extreme example of this is the autoimmune deficiency syndrome (AIDS), in which the incidence of Kaposi's sarcoma and infections with opportunistic microorganisms is relatively high because of a lack of helper T-lymphocytes.[14-16]

The "suppressor" T-lymphocyte, also called the suppressor T cell or T8-lymphocyte, helps to prevent the macrophages and other white blood cells from adversely affecting normal body cells. The proper number of T8-lymphocytes is essential. Immune homeostasis is dependent on a delicate balance of the T4/T8 ratio at 1.8:1 to 2:1.[3, 12, 17-19] A ratio below 1.8:1 or above 2:1 can predispose to autoimmune diseases such as systemic lupus erythematosus, hemolytic anemia, multiple sclerosis, severe atopic eczema, inflammatory bowel disease, and glomerulonephritis.[8, 10-13, 17, 19, 20-22]

The T-lymphocyte percent of total lymphocytes does not vary more than 10%, and rarely more than 5%, in an 8-week period.* Therefore, the measurement of T-lymphocyte percent of total lymphocytes before and after the insertion and removal of dental amalgam and nickel-base alloys can be compared with previous T-lymphocyte data to help determine biocompatibility.

PATIENT TESTS

Patient No. 1 was a 21-year-old asymptomatic white woman with no significant medical history. Dental history and examination revealed six amalgam restorations and two incipient carious lesions (Figs. 1 and 2).

Before removal of the dental amalgam, 47% of the lymphocytes were T-lymphocytes. After removal of the dental amalgam and insertion of ethyl methacrylate provisional restorations (Figs. 3 and 4), 73% of the lymphocytes were T-lymphocytes. The change from 47% to 73% represents an increase of 55.3%.

After reinsertion of four amalgam restorations (Dispersalloy, Johnson and Johnson Dental Products Co., East Windsor, N.J.) (Fig. 5), 55% of the lymphocytes were T-lymphocytes. The change from 73% to 55% represents a decrease of 24.7%.

After removal of the provisional and amalgam restorations and cementation of the eight cast gold restorations (Modulay, Jelenko Dental Health Products, Armonk, N.Y.) with silicophosphate cement (Fluorothin, S. S. White Dental Products International, Philadelphia, Pa.) (Figs. 6 and 7), 72% of the lymphocytes were T-lymphocytes. The change from 55% to 72% represents an increase of 30.9%.

Patient No. 2 was a 20-year-old asymptomatic white man with no significant medical history. Dental history

Presented at the American Prosthodontic Society, Newport Beach, Calif.

*Clinical Associate Professor, Department of Restorative Dentistry.

*Portero, J. K., SmithKline Laboratory: Personal communication, 1983.

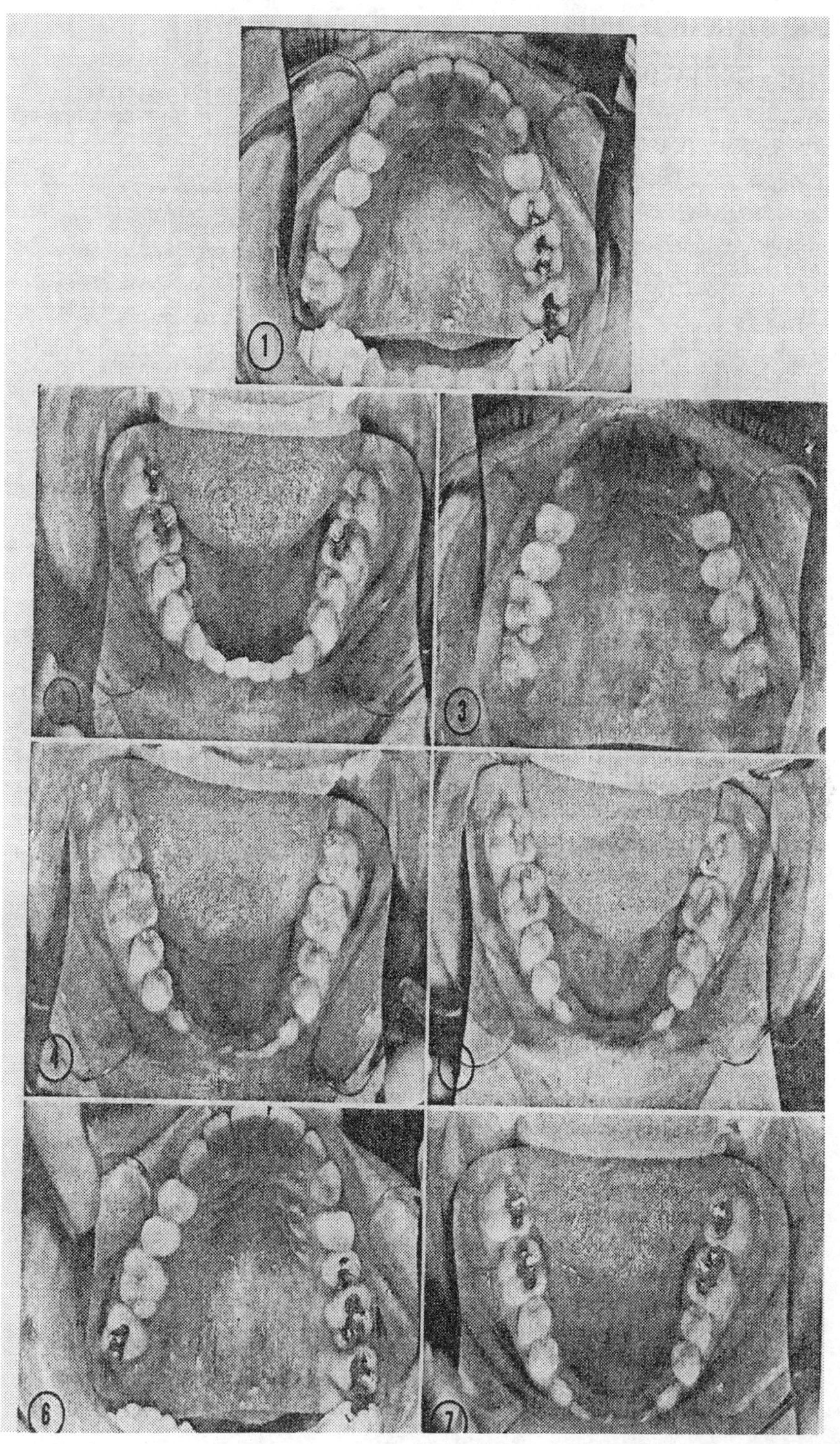
1
3
4
6
7

and examination revealed one pin-retained (TMS, Whaledent, New York, N.Y.) composite resin restoration on the maxillary right central incisor. No other dental restorations were present (Fig. 8).

Before removal of the pin-retained composite restoration, 63% of the lymphocytes were T-lymphocytes. After the pin-retained composite resin restoration was replaced with a porcelain-fused-to-nickel–base alloy (Ceramalloy II [72% nickel, beryllium free], Ceramco, Inc., East Windsor, N.J.) (Fig. 9), 56% of the lymphocytes were T-lymphocytes. The change from 63% to 56% represents a decrease of 11.1%.

After removal of the porcelain-fused-to-nickel base alloy and placement of a porcelain-fused-to-ceramic crown (Cerestore, Johnson and Johnson Dental Products) (Fig. 10), 77% of the lymphocytes were T-lymphocytes. The change from 56% to 77% represents an increase of 37.5%.

Patient No. 3 was a 35-year-old white woman. Significant medical history included advanced symptoms of multiple sclerosis. Dental history and examination revealed nine amalgam restorations (Figs. 11 and 12).

Before removal of the dental amalgam, 60% of the lymphocytes were T-lymphocytes. After removal of the dental amalgam and insertion of gold restorations (Jel-"O", Jelenko Dental Health Products) with silicophosphate cement (Fluorothin) (Figs. 13 and 14), 71% of the lymphocytes were T-lymphocytes. The change from 60% to 71% represents an increase of 18.3%.

COMMENTS

Dental amalgam and nickel alloys have been considered relatively safe based on research and clinical observation over many years.[23-34] Nevertheless, any chemical or dental material used for people must be subjected to new immunologic procedures as they become available.

Diagnosing the etiologic factors associated with an autoimmune disease is hindered by the delayed response of the immune system, the gradual onset of symptoms, and the presence of symptoms distant from the site of sensitization. Many reports of allergic reaction to dental amalgam describe a lack of oral manifestation.[24, 26, 29, 35-56] The dermatitis and urticaria associated with nickel sensitivity is most often found distant from the nickel source. The hands, neck, and eyelids are the most common areas of dermatitis and urticaria, regardless of the location of the sensitizing nickel alloy.[33, 52, 57-85]

Nickel is a known carcinogen. Industrial exposure to nickel dust and implantation of nickel alloys will markedly increase the incidence of cancer.[33, 79, 86-111] Dental technicians must be informed of the hazard of inhaling nickel grindings.

The carcinogenic potential of nickel-base dental alloys to the patient is unknown, but corrosion of nickel alloys and release of nickel ions occur with all nickel-base alloys.[33, 52, 63, 69-71, 74, 81, 83, 103, 112-122]

An abnormal T-lymphocyte percent of lymphocytes or a malfunction of T-lymphocytes can increase the risk of cancer, infectious diseases, and autoimmune diseases.[3, 8, 10-16, 19-22, 81, 83, 123] Further research is being conducted to help determine the incidence and magnitude of T-lymphocyte reduction and alteration by dental materials.

SUMMARY

Preliminary data suggest that dental amalgam and dental nickel alloys can adversely affect the quantity of T-lymphocytes.

Human T-lymphocytes can recognize specific antigens, execute effector functions, and regulate the type and intensity of virtually all cellular and humoral immune responses. Normal immune function depends on a proper quantity, quality, and ratio of T-lymphocyte helper and suppressor subsets.

Further research may determine the frequency and magnitude of T-lymphocyte reduction and alteration by dental materials.

REFERENCES

1. Guyton, A. C.: Function of the Human Body, ed 2. Philadelphia, 1964, W. B. Saunders Co., p. 94.
2. Reinherz, E. L., and Schlossman, S. F.: Regulation of the immune response—Inducer and suppressor T-lymphocyte subsets in human beings. N Engl J Med 303:370, 1980.
3. Aiuti, F., and Pandolfi, F.: The role of T lymphocytes in the

Figs. 1 and 2. Amalgam restorations in patient No. 1 before treatment. First blood test was made at this time.

Figs. 3 and 4. Acrylic resin provisional restorations in patient No. 1 after original amalgam was removed. Second blood test was made 4 weeks after placement of the restorations.

Fig. 5. Amalgam reinserted into provisional restorations in patient No. 1. Third blood test was made 4 weeks after placement of the amalgam restorations.

Figs. 6 and 7. Cast gold restorations in patient No. 1. Fourth blood test was made 6 weeks after cementing gold restorations.

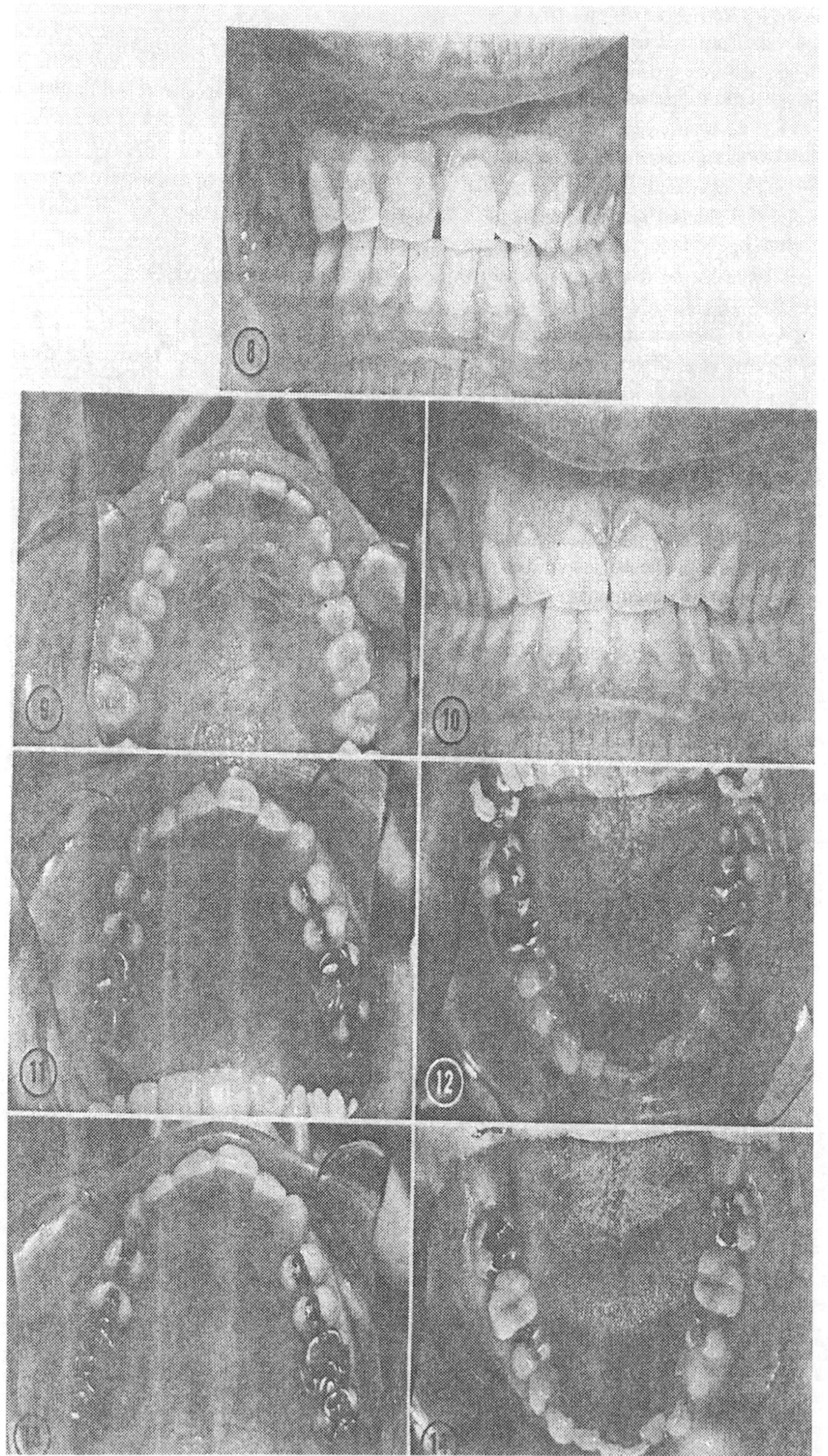
8
9
10
11
12

pathogenesis of primary immunodeficiencies. Thymus 4:257, 1982.
4. Legler, D. W., Arnold, R. R., Lynch D. P., and McGhee, J. R.: Immunodeficiency disease and implications for dental treatment. J Am Dent Assoc 105:803, 1982.
5. Noce, P. S., Ortega, P. R., and Suffin, S. C.: Immune Deficiency Report. Woodland Hills, Calif., 1984, SmithKline Clinical Laboratories, Inc., p 1.
6. Moretta, L., Mingari, M. C., and Moretta, A.: Human T cell subpopulations in normal and pathologic conditions. Immunol Rev 45:163, 1979.
7. Reinherz, E. L., and Schlossman, S. F.: The differentiation and function of human T lymphocytes. Cell 19:821, 1980.
8. Stingl, G., Gazze, L. A., Czarnecki, N., and Wolff, K.: T cell abnormalities in atopic dermatitis patients: Imbalances in T cell subpopulations and impaired generation of Con A-induced suppressor cells. J Invest Dermatol 76:468, 1981.
9. Thomas, Y., Rogozinski, L., Irigoyen, O. H., Friedman, S. M., Kung, P. C., Goldstein, G., and Chess, L.: Functional analysis of human T cell subsets defined by monoclonal antibodies. IV. Induction of suppressor cells within the OKT4+ population. J Exp Med 154:459, 1981.
10. Chatenoud, L., and Bach, M. A.: Abnormalities of T-cell subsets in glomerulonephritis and systemic lupus erythematosus. Kidney Int 20:267, 1981.
11. Frazer, I. H., and MacKay, I. R.: T lymphocyte subpopulations defined by two sets of monoclonal antibodies in chronic active hepatitis and systemic lupus erythematosus. Clin Exp Immunol 50:107, 1982.
12. Cagnoli, L., Tabacchi, P., Pasquali, S., Cenci, M., Sasdelli, M., and Zucchelli, P.: T cell subset alterations in idiopathic glomerulonephritis. Clin Exp Immunol 50:70, 1982.
13. Traugott, U., Reinherz, E. L., and Raine, C. S.: Multiple sclerosis: Distribution of T cell subsets within active chronic lesions. Science 219:308, 1983.
14. Oleske, J., Minnefor, A., Cooper, Jr., R., Thomas, K., dela Cruz, A., Ahdieh, H., Guerrero, I., Joshi, V. V., and Desposito, F.: Immune deficiency syndrome in children. J Am Med Assoc 249:2345, 1983.
15. Rubinstein, A., Sicklick, M., Gupta, A., Bernstein, L., Klein, N., Rubinstein, E., Spigland, I., Fruchter, L., Litman, N., Lee, H., and Hollander, M.: Acquired immunodeficiency with reversed T4/T8 ratios in infants born to promiscuous and drug-addicted mothers. J Am Med Assoc 249:2350, 1983.
16. Sonnabend, J., Witkin, S. S., and Purtilo, D. T.: Acquired immunodeficiency syndrome, opportunistic infections, and malignancies in male homosexuals. J Am Med Assoc 249:2370, 1983.
17. Leung, D. Y. M., Rhodes, A. R., and Geha, R. S.: Enumeration of T cell subsets of atopic dermatitis using monoclonal antibodies. J Allergy Clin Immunol 67:450, 1981.
18. Faure, M. R., Gaucherand, M. A., Thivolet, J., Czernielewski, J. M., and Nicolas, J. F.: Decreased levels of T-cells and cells with suppressor T-cell phenotype as defined by specific monoclonal antibodies in patients with atopic dermatitis. Clin Exp Dermatol 7:513, 1982.
19. Butler, M., Atherton, D., and Levinsky, R. J.: Quantitiative and functional deficit of suppressor T cells in children with atopic eczema. Clin Exp Immunol 50:92, 1982.
20. Reinherz, E. L., Weiner, H. L., Hauser, S. L., Cohen, J. A., Distaso, J. A., and Schlossman, S. F.: Loss of suppressor T cells in active multiple sclerosis. N Engl J Med 303:125, 1980.
21. Morimoto, C., Reinherz, E. L., Schlossman, S. F., Schur, P. H., Mills, J. A., and Steinberg, A. D.: Alterations in immunoregulatory T cell subsets in active systemic lupus erythematosus. J Clin Invest 66:1171, 1980.
22. Kohler, P. F., and Vaughn, J.: The autoimmune diseases. J Am Med Assoc 248:2446, 1982.
23. Hoover, A. W., and Goldwater, L. J.: Absorption and excretion of mercury in man—X. Dental amalgams as a source of urinary mercury. Arch Environ Health 12:506, 1966.
24. Shovelton, D. S.: Silver amalgam and mercury allergy. Oral Surg 25:29, 1968.
25. Rupp, N. W., and Paffenbarger, G. C.: Significance to health of mercury used in dental practice: A review. J Am Dent Assoc 82:1401, 1971.
26. Craig, R., and Peyton, F., editors: Restorative Dental Materials, ed 5. St. Louis, 1975, The C. V. Mosby Co., pp 169-182, 203-204.
27. Barolet, R. Y.: Mercury: The unseen hazard in the dental office. Dent Student 56:62, 1977.
28. Carrel, R., Mackowiak, E. D., Chialastri, A. J., and Binns, W. H.: Accumulation of the base metals (copper, zinc and mercury) in human body. J Dent Child 46:30, 1979.
29. Jendresen, M. D.: Mercury in dental amalgam: Is it safe? J Calif Dent Assoc 10:31, 1982.
30. Hansen, L. S., and Silverman, Jr., S.: Localized tissue reaction to implanted amalgam: A review. J Calif Dent Assoc 10:33, 1982.
31. Bauer, J. G., and First, H. A.: The toxicity of mercury in dental amalgam. J Calif Dent Assoc 10:47, 1982.
32. American Dental Association Council on Dental Materials, Instruments, and Equipment and the American Dental Association Council on Dental Therapeutics: Safety of dental amalgam. J Am Dent Assoc 106:519, 1983.
33. American Dental Association Council on Dental Materials, Instruments, and Equipment: Biological effects of nickel-

Fig. 8. Pin-retained composite restoration on patient No. 2 before treatment. First blood test was made at this time.

Fig. 9. Porcelain-fused-to-nickel–base alloy crown in patient No. 2 after removal of pin and composite resin. Second blood test was made 6 weeks after cementing crown.

Fig. 10. Porcelain-ceramic crown in patient No. 2 after removal of porcelain-fused-to-nickel–base alloy crown. Third blood test was made 6 weeks after cementing restoration.

Figs. 11 and **12.** Amalgam restorations in patient No. 3 before treatment. First blood test was made at this time.

Figs. 13 and **14.** Gold restorations in patient No. 3. Second blood test was made 6 months after cementing gold restorations.

containing dental alloys. J Am Dent Assoc **104**:501, 1982.
34. Moffa, J. P., Ellison, J. E., and Hamilton, J. C.: Incidence of nickel sensitivity in dental patients. Am Assoc Dent Res **62**:199, 1983 (Abstr No. 271).
35. Markow, H.: Urticaria following a dental silver filling—Case report. NY State J Med **43**:1648, 1943.
36. Bass, M. H.: Idiosyncrasy to metallic mercury, with special reference to amalgam fillings in the teeth. J Pediatr **23**:215, 1943.
37. Robinson, H. M., and Bereston, E. S.: Contact dermatitis due to the mercury of amalgam dental fillings. Arch Dermatol Syph **59**:116, 1949.
38. Johnson, H. H., Schonberg, I. L., and Bach, N. F.: Chronic atopic dermatitis, with pronounced mercury sensitivity: Partial clearing after extraction of teeth containing mercury amalgam fillings. Arch Dermatol Syph **63**:279, 1951.
39. Spector, L. A.: Allergic manifestation to mercury. J Am Dent Assoc **42**:320, 1951.
40. Goldwater, L. J.: The toxicology of inorganic mercury. Ann NY Acad Sci **65**:498, 1957.
41. Fernstrom, A. I. B., Frykholm, K. O., and Huldt, S.: Mercury allergy with eczematous dermatitis due to silver amalgam fillings. Br Dent J **113**:204, 1962.
42. Engelman, M. A.: Mercury allergy resulting from amalgam restorations. J Am Dent Assoc **66**:122, 1963.
43. Bergenholtz, A.: Multiple polypous hyperplasias of the oral mucosa with regression after removal of amalgam fillings. Acta Odontol Scand **23**:111, 1965.
44. Gaul, L. E.: Immunity of the oral mucosa in epidermal sensitization to mercury. Arch Dermatol **93**:45, 1966.
45. Strassburg, M., and Schubel, K.: Generalisierte allergischen Reaktion durch Silberamalgamfüllungen. Dtsch Zahnarztl Z **22**:3, 1967.
46. Juhlin, L., and Ohman, S.: Allergic reaction to mercury in red tattoos and mucosa adjacent to amalgam fillings. Acta Derm Venereol (Stockh) **48**:103, 1968.
47. Witek, E.: A case of hypersensitivity to mercury released from amalgam fillings. Czas Stomatol **22**:311, 1968.
48. Frykholm, K. O., Frithiof, L., Fernstrom, A. I. B., Moberger, G., Blohm, S. G., and Bjorn, E.: Allergy to copper derived from dental alloys as a possible cause of oral lesions of lichen planus. Acta Derm Venereol (Stockh) **49**:268, 1969.
49. Djerassi, E., and Berova, N.: The possibilities of allergic reactions from silver amalgam restorations. Int Dent J **19**:481, 1969.
50. Thomson, J., and Russell, J.: Dermatitis due to mercury following amalgam dental restorations. Br J Dermatol **82**:292, 1970.
51. Wright, F.: Allergic reaction to mercury after dental treatment. NZ Dent J **67**:251, 1971.
52. Fisher, A. A., and Frazier, C. A., editors: Dentistry and the Allergic Patient. Springfield, Ill, 1970, Charles C Thomas Publisher, chap 10.
53. Feuerman, E.: Dermatitis due to mercury in amalgam dental fillings. Contact Dermatitis **1**:191, 1975.
54. Feuerman, E.: Recurrent contact dermatitis caused by mercury in amalgam dental fillings. Int J Dermatol **14**:657, 1975.
55. Soremark, R., Mishah, D., and Arvidson, K.: Autoradiographic study of distribution patterns of metals which occur as corrosion products from dental restorations. Scand J Dent Res 87:450, 1979.
56. Hanzely, B., and Hadhazy, S.: Allergic reaction elicited by amalgam filling. Fogorv Sz **73**:208, 1980.
57. Gaul, L. E.: Metal sensitivity in eczema of the hands. Ann Allergy **11**:758, 1953.
58. Fisher, A. A., and Shapiro, A.: Allergic eczematous contact dermatitis due to metallic nickel. J Am Med Assoc **161**:717, 1956.
59. Calnan, C. D.: Nickel dermatitis. Br J Dermatol **68**:229, 1956.
60. Calnan, C. D.: Nickel sensitivity in women. Int Arch Allergy Appl Immunol **11**:73, 1957.
61. Foussereau, J., and Laugier, P.: Allergic eczemas from metallic foreign bodies. Clin Dermatologica **52**:221, 1966.
62. Gaul, L. E.: Development of allergic nickel dermatitis from earring. J Am Med Assoc **200**:176, 1967.
63. Boyanov, B., Popov, K., Todorov, I., and Ekimov, B.: Experimental electro-chemical and biological tests on some dental materials. Int Dent J **18**:421, 1968.
64. Brendlinger, D. L., and Tarsitano, J. J.: Generalized dermatitis due to sensitivity to a chrome-cobalt removable partial denture. J Am Dent Assoc **81**:392, 1970.
65. Tinckler, L. F.: Nickel sensitivity to surgical skin clips. Br J Surg **59**:745, 1972.
66. Barranco, V. P., and Soloman, H.: Eczematous dermatitis from nickel (letter). J Am Med Assoc **220**:1244, 1972.
67. McNeely, M. D., Nechay, M. W., and Sunderman, Jr., F. W.: Measurements of nickel in serum and urine as indices of environmental exposure to nickel. Clin Chem **18**:992, 1972.
68. Barranco, V. P., and Soloman, H.: Eczematous dermatitis caused by internal exposure to nickel. South Med J **66**:447, 1973.
69. Speer, F., and Dockhorn, A.: Allergy and Immunology in Childhood. Springfield, Ill, 1973, Charles C Thomas, Publisher, pp 297-298, 535.
70. Samitz, M. H., and Klein, A.: Nickel dermatitis hazards from prosthesis. (Letter to the Editor) J Am Med Assoc **223**:1159, 1973.
71. Fisher, A.: Contact Dermatitis, ed. 2. Philadelphia, 1973, Lea & Febiger, chaps 1, 4, and 6.
72. Wood, J. F.: Mucosal reaction to cobalt-chromium alloy. Br Dent J **136**:423, 1974.
73. Levantine, A. V., and Bettley, F. R.: Sensitivity to metal dental plate. Proc R Soc Med **67**:1007, 1974.
74. Schriver, W. R., Shereff, R. H., Domnitz, J. M., Swintak, E. F., and Civjan, S.: Allergic response to stainless steel wire. Oral Surg **42**:578, 1976.
75. Moffa, J. P., Beck, W. D., and Hoke, A. W.: Allergic response to nickel containing dental alloys. J Dent Res **56**(Special issue B):78 (Abstr No. 107) 1977.
76. Wahs, P. L., and Spruit, D.: Course of nickel contact dermatitis. Contact Dermatitis **5**:57, 1979.
77. Peltonen, L.: Nickel sensitivity in the general population. Contact Dermatitis **5**:27, 1979.
78. Prystowsky, S. D.: Allergic contact hypersensitivity to nickel, neomycin, ethylenediamine and benzocaine. Arch Dermatol **115**:959, 1979.
79. McNail, E. G.: Prevailing evidence shows nickel alloys cause cancer. Dent Lab World **6**:25, 1979.
80. Bergman, M., Bergman, B., and Soremark, R.: Tissue accumulation of nickel released due to electrochemical corrosion of non-precious dental casting alloys. J Oral Rehabil **7**:325, 1980.
81. Newman, S., Chamberlain, R. T., and Nunez, L. J.: Nickel solubility from nickel-chromium dental casting alloys. J Biomed Mater Res **15**:615, 1981.

Dr. Harold Kristal, D.D.S., also completed a thirty-case study checking the immune panels to see the effect of metals on patient's health. A fact of crucial importance is that the immune system made a dramatic change after the metals had been removed. Metals depress the immune system.

Important point: stainless steel wires used in orthodontics and base metals in crowns and bridges usually contain nickel. Dentistry commonly uses metals containing toxic nickel for crowns with porcelain baked to this metal making the crown look like a normal tooth.

An Orthodontic Wire Story

Orthodontic wires contain nickel and can cause personality changes. One mother said her children did not hug and kiss her as they did before they had acquired braces. She also noticed a lowering of their grade point average and the children no longer helped around the house. A homeopathic remedy for nickel was made for each child. Within two days the children returned to their pre-braces personality, grades went up and hugs and kisses became the norm.

Chapter 9

Root Canal Treatments ("Root Canals") May Adversely Affect Your Health

Let us carefully define what the phrase "root canal" means; actually this has two possible meanings: one of them is the part of a tooth's structure, known as the root canal; the second meaning refers to "root canal treatment" of a tooth, which is called a "root canal" for short, with the word "treatment" left off.

The part of the tooth known as the "root canal" is the soft inner portion of the tooth, inside the root (or roots, if the tooth has more than one root). The roots of the tooth are the portions of the tooth that extend into the jaw bone and are anchored with small ligaments into the jaw or socket that holds the tooth. The roots of a tooth are important for feeding the tooth just as the roots of a tree are important to nourish the tree. A normal tooth is a living organ and inside the visible part of the tooth (the "crown") is a soft portion, at the very inside, called the pulp chamber. This pulp chamber holds blood, lymph vessels and nerves; cells line the wall of the pulp chamber to feed the little tunnel that nourish the dentine of the tooth. The soft pulp part of the tooth has extensions going down into each root of the tooth, and these soft insides of the root are the root canals.

When a tooth has died, something drastic has to be done to deal with the health threat of a decaying and increasingly toxic dead tooth. The options are only two 1) extract the tooth or 2) "save" the tooth by cleaning out all of the soft inside parts – the pulp chamber and the root canals (not missing any of them), sterilizing it thoroughly, and filling the pulp chamber and all root canals with some anti-microbial milling materials to try to keep the tooth sterile and infection-free forever. This latter procedure is called "root canal treatment" of the tooth and, somewhat confusingly, a tooth that has been so treated is called a "root canal." It would be more correct to call it a "root canalled tooth," or, even better, a "root canal treated tooth."

But the root canal treated tooth may not be trouble-free forever. Even if the tooth is pretty well sterilized at root canal treatment time, they tend to become infected, over time. Those infections often become extremely toxic, with a predominance of anaerobic bacteria (the extremely toxic ones that thrive in the absence of oxygen) and fungi. Tests done at ALT, Inc. show that about 25% of the root canalled teeth tested there are "extremely toxic," another 50% of root canalled teeth tested are "toxic." Only about 25% of them are tested as "not very toxic." So, the odds are not very good that life with a root canal treated tooth will be trouble free; and the more of these treated teeth that you have, the greater the likelihood that some of them will be toxic or extremely toxic; such toxic teeth may give you symptoms in a remote part of your body – but probably on the tooth's meridian – such as heart disease, breast cancer or some other cancer, arthritic symptoms, etc. An examining physician is unlikely to use CEDS or any other tool to link a root canal treated tooth or teeth to the chronic health condition that is bringing the patient into the clinic.

More locally, the toxic root canal tooth may well produce an abscess next to its root or roots and also jawbone infection, which may add to the symptoms and health problems that conventional medicine often, has such a hard time finding the cause of a health problem. Like toxic, infected root canal treated teeth, jawbone cavitations may cause pain and perhaps chronic illness for a long time before the real cause is discovered – if it ever is discovered.

Let me tell you about a well-known root canal procedure, and how thousands of root canals are performed every working day on unsuspecting patients. Your body does not like infection or dead tissue of any kind, much less an infection from a root canal. Every organ and tissue system is directly affected by healthy teeth as well as teeth that are dead. Reading case histories in this book will help you understand the importance of having natural healthy teeth and removing teeth that are not healthy.

I like the statement a dentist made when I said; "I would rather lose a tooth than a body function." Another dentist said, "I would rather die than lose a tooth." I said, "You will if you keep infected teeth. Remember all root canals are infected."

Consider this: No dead tooth is worth saving if it will cause the loss of a body function. Look at the Energetic Relations of Teeth (odontons) with respect to Organ and Tissue Systems chart (Teeth and Body Energy Chart).

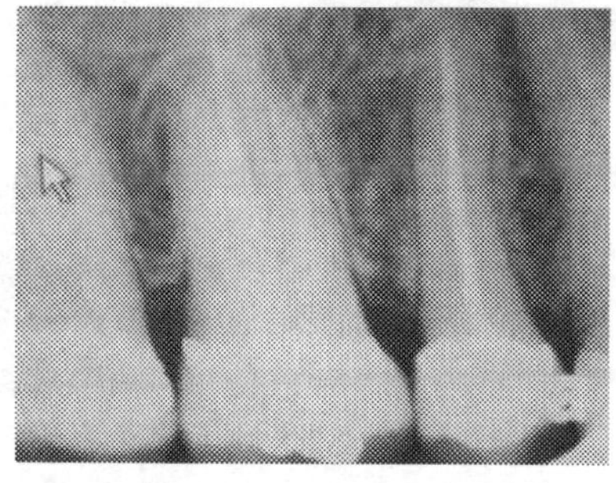

Refer to the Teeth Body Energy Chart, the upper second bicuspids are related to the large intestine and lung; the upper first molar is related to the stomach, spleen and pancreas, thyroid, parathyroid, and maxillary sinus. Most root canals are filled with Gutta Percha, which usually contains cadmium salts, a heavy toxic metal. Cadmium is a toxic metal which tends to cause high blood pressure, and which will exacerbate the toxicity of any mercury present in the body. Whether root canal treated teeth are filled with Gutta Percha or with calcium-based fillers, neither can overcome past infection nor protect the tooth from new infection.

See the following articles for more information on the effects of cadmium:

Waalker, M.P., Rehm, S., Cadmium and prostate cancer, *J Toxicological Environmental Health*, 43:251-269, 1994

Coogan, T.P., Bare, R.M., Waalker, M.P., Cadmium-induced DNA damage: Effects of zinc pretreatment, *Toxicological Applied Pharmaceuticals*, 113:227-233, 1992

Heath, J.C., Daniel, I.R., Webb, M., et al, Cadmium as a carcinogen, *Nature*, 193:592-593, 1962

Remember: It is the energy and physical substance of restorative dental materials that can be a toxic burden to our health. You can get a MSDS (Material Safety Data Sheet) on Gutta Percha from your dental products supplier representative.

Remember again that everything is energy; dental material energy not compatible with your energy can make the difference between health and sickness. Most root canal filled teeth have a number of different materials in them, on them, or around them. You already know about the electrical effect of metals on the hard tissue (teeth and bone) and soft tissue (gum, tongue and cheeks). Refer to chapter 3 for review of electrical effect of metals; also refer to reference section for chapters 3 and 9 for additional information.

Example: A root canal treated molar I extracted had a stainless steel (toxic with nickel) crown on the tooth covering a mercury silver amalgam filling (causing a strong battery effect). In these root canals were silver points, gutta percha points, and a cementing material around those inserted points, making this a toxic, abscessed tooth.

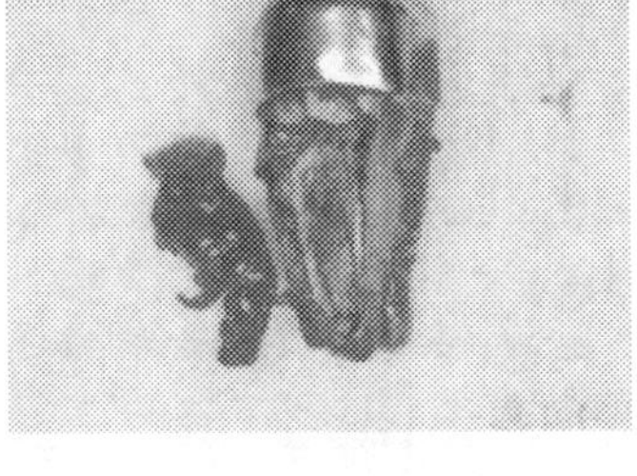

The abscess is on the left of the root canal treated tooth.

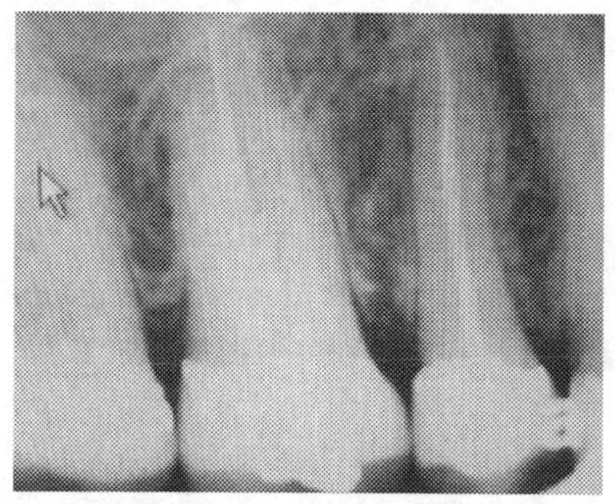

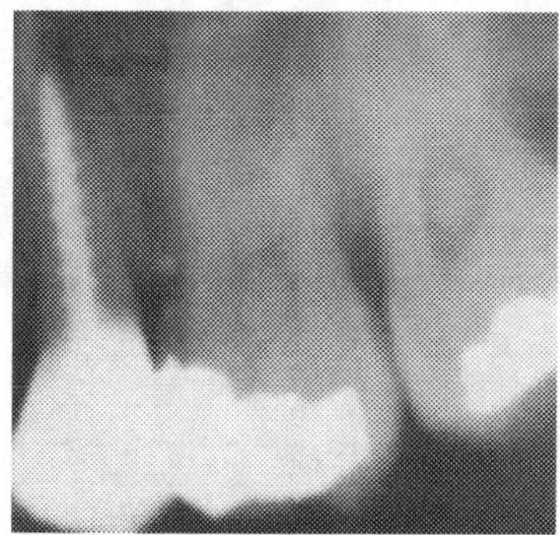

Adding to the energy problem of these teeth is a metal filling, and root canal causing various symptoms, often overlooked.

Visualizing a Nerve

Envision a weed pulled from the ground with its main taproot and the auxiliary root fibers attached; the nerve in a tooth looks like this, with tiny branches of nerve fibers coming off the main nerve. Main nerves you can see on an x-ray but the tiny branches do not show. Infection can be found any place along the root. Rotting small nerve fibers that cannot be filled or lasered produce a poison that will be the start of an infected tooth.

Dentists can only see and work with the main root canal to clean out the infection. They cannot see the many small nerves inside the dentine roots. These "accessory" canals are so thin they cannot be filled; therefore continuing to promote an abscess. Dr. Boyd Haley, Professor of Chemistry, and Toxicologist at the University of Kentucky, states, "All root canals are infected." See the Teeth and Body Energy chart for any root canal tooth location in your oral cavity to see how it could affect your health.

You can also go to: www.iaomt.com for root canal information.

Refer to Dr. Volls Book: *Interrelations of Odontons And Tonsils To Organs, Fields Of Disturbance, And Tissue Systems*. Order from www.vibranthealth.com

Root Canal Cover Up Exposed! by Dr. George Meinig, DDS,

Weston Price's work on root canals is found at Price Pottenger foundation, www.price-pottenger.org.

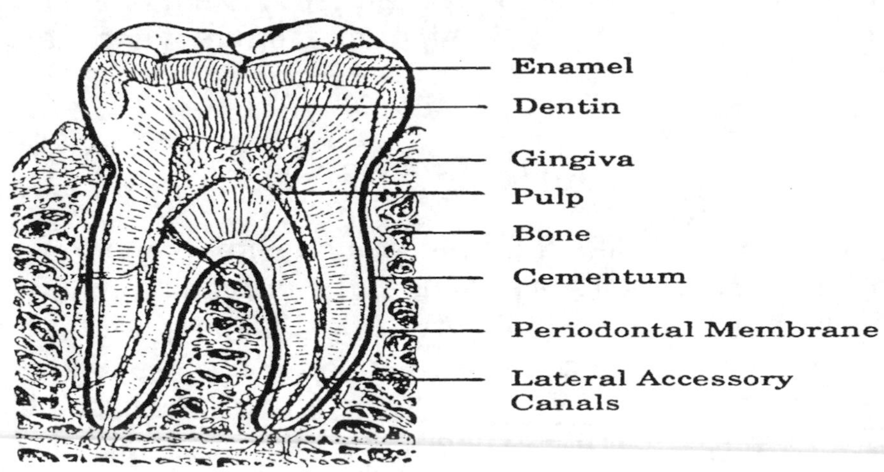

Note lateral accessory canals.

Chapter 10

Replacing Missing Teeth

An implant is a burden to the health in two ways:

First, there is no compatible implant material that checks out well with CEDS. On the other hand mechanical implants are helpful in holding a denture in place. Side effects of implant materials may take days or years to produce physical or mental health problems.

A second disadvantage is the gingival (gum tissue) fluid around the implant. This gingival fluid may contain a bacterial and protein toxin that spreads throughout the entire system of the patient. A TOPAS test indicates the toxicity of the fluid around the implant. The TOPAS test is a very simple, non-invasive technique developed by Dr. Boyd Haley, who acknowledges any amount of toxin is poisonous to a patient's health.

The TOPAS TEST: for the dentist

Follow the directions closely by placing a chemically free paper point under the free margin of the gum at the neck of the implant or root canal tooth for one minute. This test paper is then placed in a test fluid, in a colorimeter (a form of spectrometer but measures a set wave length) that reads the toxins in this fluid. There is no such thing as a little bit of poison, you are either being poisoned or you are not, and a TOPAS test will tell.

Dr. Haley changed the chemistry of the test fluid to make it more sensitive. It measures the level of reactive thiols which are found in the mouth only if anaerobic bacteria cause them to be there. These are hydrogen sulfide (H2S), and methylthiol or mercaptan (CH3-SH) (bad breath).

You can find references on implants at www.iaomt.com. The improved TOPAS II test is Halitox instrument and kit information for measuring hydrogen sulfide (rotten eggs smell) in the oral cavity.

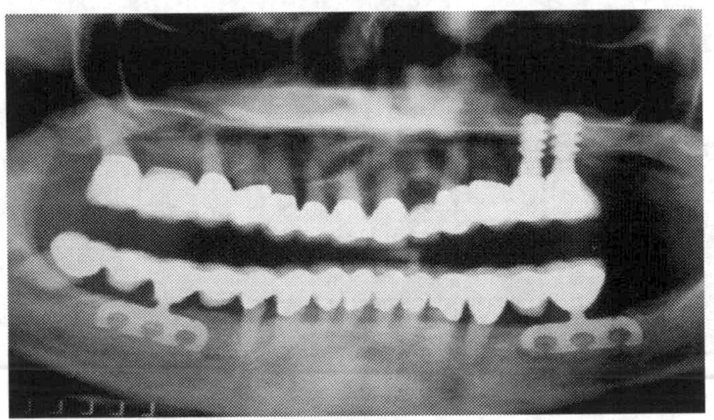

X-ray of dental implants

Denture Materials:

Standard denture acrylics or plastics used in making dentures have a pink color made with a cadmium metal oxide. On the other hand the compatible plastic I use, Vitalon 1060, is cadmium free. It is made by Fricke International (phone # 800-539-4253) in the USA. Partial dentures that are flexible are made with a chemical many patients cannot tolerate. CEDS can check for compatibility with the patient, as plastics used in dentures and partials, if not compatible, they can cause health problems.

Lab Information for Dentists:

Cook Dental Lab processes the denture to the finished hard plastic with a hot water curing method using 167 degrees for 20 hours. Other laboratories use other methods, curing with a light and injection molding to harden the denture plastics. I like the twenty-hour hot water cure to remove the monomer (monomer is the liquid used in making the denture base) making the denture as compatible as possible with this technique.

Everyone has a different degree of sensitivity. We in the dental profession must make every effort to help these sensitive patients.

A Temporary

Covering a tooth, once it has been prepared to make an inlay, crown, or bridge is called a temporary restoration. A function of temporary filling materials is to protect the tooth while the permanent restoration is being made. Care must be taken to use compatible temporary materials, and a good example is the use of aluminum in temporary crowns. Aluminum has a high electrical charge that causes pain. Beware of inexpensive metal and plastic temporaries, their energy or chemical fumes, can make patients ill.

For a list of the most compatible temporary materials refer to chapter 16, dental material section.

Information for the dentist: Durelon cement by 3M ESPE is one of the best cements for bonding the temporaries to the tooth.

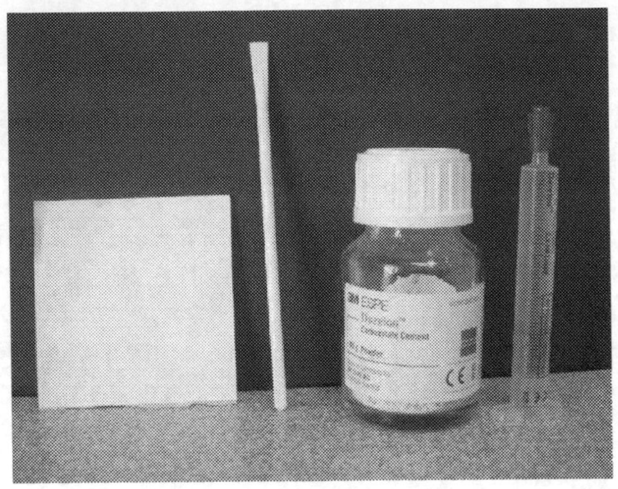

To order Durelon Cement contact:

Dental Health Products Inc.
2614 North Sugar Bush Rd
P.O. Box 176
New Franken, WI 54229-1076
1-800-626-2163
Or call your local dealer.

Chapter 11

Fluoride: A Neurotoxin

Studies done by Dr. Phylis Mulenix, Ph.D. and Robert Isaacson, Ph.D. prove without a doubt that fluoride is a neurotoxin. Toothpaste with fluoride is toxic for both children and adults. Fluoride is an enzyme and hormone inhibitor, affecting the nervous system as well as digestion. Fluoride is the major cause of brittle bones and teeth. Fluoride is the main cause of mottled enamel, producing white, light gray or brown spots on the teeth.

References: *Fluoride: the Aging Factor*, By Dr. John Yiamonuyiannis ISBN 0-913571-01-6 This book is available at libraries.

Go to chapter 11 references for the toxic fluoride connection found in most composites.

(Benagiano, A., (1965). The effect of sodium fluoride on thyroid enzymes and basal metabolism in the rat. *Annali Di Stomatologia*. Vol. 13, pp. 601-619.)

(Stolc, V., and Podoba, J., (1960). Effect of fluoride on the biogenesis of thyroid hormones. *Nature*. Vol. 188, No. 4753, pp. 855-856.)

In Dr. Sherry Rogers' book *Detoxify or Die*, you can find fluoride on pages 19, 21, 22. To find more information go to www.fluoride-free-dentistry.com or paul@flouridealert.org

Chapter 12

Tooth And Jaw Case Histories

The oral cavity is an important part of a health exam. Two patients came to me directly from the hospital after being released with broken jaws that their physician had over looked. Both patients had to be referred to an oral surgeon who set their jaws. Hidden jaw infections, as well as fractures of teeth and jaws are key factors in every health evaluation if a patient is going to become well.

An important spot in the oral cavity is the ninth space, directly behind the wisdom tooth. Dr. Voll referred to this ninth space as a possible health problem to the same organ and tissue systems affected by the wisdom teeth. Remember Dr. Voll's statement: 80 to 90 % of systemic problems are caused or influenced by the oral cavity.

Case: Jerome, age 79, ninth space

Dr. Stone referred Jerome, a 79 year-old man with heart pain, to our office. Jerome had all of his wisdom teeth. Remembering what Dr. Voll said about the ninth space, I followed his advice and found infection in the upper right space behind his wisdom tooth with the CEDS and removed the infection. Dr. Stone checked Jerome eight to ten weeks after healing, and sent me a report, stating that Jerome was pain free and feeling good. We must be aware of these hidden areas in the jaws, especially when all other points in the oral cavity look healthy.

Wisdom teeth exert an influence on many of the body's systems: the central nervous system, limbic system (mental attitude), heart, small intestine, kidney function, inner, middle, and external ear, and the tissues associated with these systems. Dr. Voll said, "one hundred percent of heart problems are related to wisdom teeth or where they were." He reminds us that the major meridians are connected throughout the entire body by secondary meridians. Bad teeth on the right side can cause problems that cross over to the left side of the body. Without knowing these relationships we are unable to find many health problems.

Case: David, age 17, depression

David had one mercury amalgam filling in his lower right first molar, and was taking anti-depressants. He was on a very good diet, and had a good home life, with caring parents. But Dr. Stone found a problem with his wisdom teeth when checking with CEDS, and advised David to have his wisdom teeth removed.

My first step was to remove that one mercury amalgam filling; after I removed the right upper and lower wisdom teeth, David's mood and mental functions quickly improved. Aware of the results from his extractions, David was very willing to have the left wisdom teeth removed on his second appointment.

Associated with the nervous system, kidneys, and the small intestine, the wisdom teeth play a major role in the mental and physical health of many patients. Be aware of this when being treated by health professionals who do not understand the oral cavity's relationship to our entire body.

Case: Dorothy, age 63, head, neck and shoulder pain, and vertigo.

Dorothy, a teacher, was unable to stand in her class room without holding on to something, and because of her serious head, neck, and shoulder pain, was rushed to a hospital for CAT and MRI scans. No physical problems could be detected.

Dorothy's retirement was two years away, and without finishing these two years her monthly retirement checks would be less. Hearing about the affect of teeth and jaws on her health, she asked me if I could help her. I detected a cavitation with CEDS in #17 (lower left wisdom tooth that was missing). I told Dorothy this would be my first cavitation surgery, she said, "Let's do it."

The bone looked healthy and solid when I opened the gum tissue. As I was cutting through the outer layer of bone the drill fell into a large, soft, green, soupy pocket, immediately indicating jawbone cavitation. Checking with CEDS after surgically removing the infected, diseased region, her jaw conductance point Ly 2, balanced perfectly, starting the healing process.

The next day Dorothy reported the pain in her head, neck and shoulder was gone. Two days later, her vertigo left, allowing her to finish her last two years of teaching and retire with full pay. A medical doctor trained in CEDS could have found the cause of Dorothy's problem.

One year later Dorothy's symptoms returned, followed by a trip to the hospital for CAT and MRI scans. She received the same report, "nothing was wrong." Dorothy immediately called me for an appointment to check her wisdom tooth area. Yes, I found the same cavitation problem that needed more surgery. Opening the very same area, I found the hole had healed almost completely with new bone. A light cleaning and closure of the gum tissue put Dorothy back on her feet to enjoy her retirement.

Case: Nick, age 58, hearing loss in one ear.

Nick, an airline pilot, had lost the hearing in his left ear. His physical was coming up, and failing it would cause him to be grounded two years before retirement. Taking a desk job would mean a decrease in his retirement pay. A patient of Dr. Stone, Nick consulted him about his hearing. Dr. Stone advised him to see an oral surgeon for removal of infection in his upper left wisdom tooth area (#16). His hearing returned immediately after the oral surgeon injected the anesthetic for surgery and cleaned that area, however that night his hearing left again. Nick called my office asking if I could help him as he was very desperate to pass his physical. The next morning I called to tell him a 10:00 am cancellation was available, and he said he would take the appointment.

Refer to the Teeth and Body Energy chart to see how upper wisdom teeth are associated with ear problems. In checking him with the CEDS, I found an area directly behind the upper left second molar that indicated possible pathology related to his hearing loss. I completed the surgery and rechecked the surgical site with CEDS, obtaining a good reading. Only after a return of his hearing would we know that the operation was successful. Nick called me that night; his hearing had returned! He was extremely happy that he would retire with full pay.

Case: Doug Cook, the author of this book, age 56, heart and jaw relationship

I use a heart monitor when I run, and set the high end heart rate at 145 beats per minute. Should the rate go higher, an alarm would go off telling me to slow down. One morning, after running 1 ½ miles, the alarm went off. The monitor showed 220 beats per minute. Immediately I started walking, and the heart slowed to its normal beat.

Good fortune was with me while attending a seminar by Dr. Andrew Landerman, D.D.S. I became aware of the relationship between the wisdom teeth and the heart. A CEDS reading of the heart and jaw, pointed directly to # 32, the lower right wisdom tooth, which had been extracted by my father when I was 16. After a jaw bone surgery at the site was performed by Dr. Landerman, I could run without a rapid heart rate.

Case: Hilda, age 41, jaw pain

Hilda had an ongoing sore throat for two years. ENT doctors and oral surgeons found no problem with the jaws, throat, ears or sinuses. Using CEDS, I checked her lower jaw where the wisdom teeth had been and found both sides to be out of balance. Surgical cleaning of these two areas brought immediate comfort to her throat. By using the CEDS it was easy to find the infection, and check the post-operative site. Biopsy reports of the jaw bone in the area of the wisdom teeth, confirmed pathology. Hilda was a thankful, pain-free patient.

Case: Mary Ann, age 24, dramatic case of vomiting.

In the fall of 1985 while having my office painted, the painter asked me about possible causes of his daughter-in-law's case of anorexia (inability to eat) and vomiting five times a day for three months. I told him it could possibly be a deficiency of zinc or the presence of electricity in her silver amalgams fillings. I sent a bottle of zinc tablets home for Mary Ann to try over the weekend. On Monday her husband told me the zinc had made no difference; Mary Ann was still vomiting and losing weight. She had lost 25 pounds over the previous three months. Her medical doctor had given her prescriptions for the vomiting with no effect, and had told Mary Ann it was all in her head. Mary Ann had made an appointment with a psychiatrist who found her mentally healthy.

I suggested we check with CEDS for any problem with her fillings. The CEDS evaluation indicated there was a body imbalance. I felt her vomiting could be caused by mercury silver amalgams fillings. Examining her teeth, I found six small fillings on the chewing surface of the molars. In one appointment, I removed all amalgam fillings and placed six non-metal oxide composites. Driving home that afternoon she told her husband she felt a sensation but did not have to vomit. Within two days after the mercury removal, Mary Ann could eat food and lead a normal life. The good results prompted her to ask if I could help her with the sore throat that she had had for five months. I checked her recent wisdom teeth extraction sites, # 17 and #32 with CEDS, and that revealed a problem, possibly related to her sore throat.

Mary Ann returned to the oral surgeon who had removed her wisdom teeth. She asked if it was possible her sore throat could be caused by the extractions. The oral surgeon told her the extractions had nothing to do with her throat problem. The removal of her fillings with good results brought her back to see if I could help her sore throat. The wisdom teeth area on the lower right and left needed only an opening of the gum tissue to change the energy field. Immediately after the anesthetic left the lower jaw, her throat pain was gone.

Their excitement with the results took Mary Ann and her husband back to their M.D. to tell him they found a cure to Mary Ann's vomiting. The medical doctor said, "You can believe that if you want to." Angrily, Mary Ann's husband said to the doctor, "I don't care if Dr. Cook would have danced around her with feathers, her vomiting stopped."

Wisdom Teeth in General

Impacted or congenitally missing wisdom teeth or the area where a wisdom tooth has been extracted can have far reaching effects on the total health of mind and body. Wisdom teeth are related to varying symptoms such as: low energy, poor mental attitude, nervousness, indigestion, rapid or irregular heart rate, hearing problems, vertigo, pain, and impaired kidney function.

All fillings must be checked for compatibility before performing oral surgery, especially in the wisdom tooth area.

Checking the site post-operatively (after surgery) with CEDS for removal of residual pathology ensures a greater prospect for good healing.

Remember, upper molars and lower bicuspids, 2, 3, 14, 15, and 20, 21, 28, 29 are all associated with the stomach, spleen and pancreas. Our energy level goes up when we are able to digest food properly.

This next case is a good example of the effect of the oral cavity on organ systems.

Case: Mrs. K, age 58, diarrhea.

Mrs. K's diarrhea, a problem of two years duration, was being caused by a large piece of amalgam filling. I saw the silver mercury filling on the x-ray, along with a dark blue color in the jaw area # 28, which is related to the pancreas. This was the first dramatic case in which I could clearly see the relationship between the first bicuspid and the pancreas, and it encouraged me to continue to investigate the relationship between health problems and the oral cavity.

Her former dentist did not see that the mercury amalgam filling had fallen into the socket during the extraction. Tissue had healed over the extraction site, making the patient think everything was normal. Mrs. K had developed this diarrhea fifteen years after the tooth had been extracted. Her medical doctor, with all his prescriptions, could not stop this torment of loose stool.

I was preparing a crown on the lower right cuspid before I was to make a partial replacing her missing posterior teeth. Right behind the cuspid is the jaw area associated with her digestive system, and is the area related to the pancreas. According to Dr. Voll, problems in this area can cause diarrhea.

Mrs. K. did not want me to remove her mercury silver amalgam until I told her about the relationship between this material and problems in the intestinal tract. Then she agreed to the removal of the mercury silver amalgam, and I placed two sutures to close the surgical opening. She returned for suture removal and proceeded to tell me what had happened to her. "I did not think I should talk over my physical problems with a dentist, but I have had diarrhea for two years. When you told me about the metal in my jaw and how it could affect my intestinal tract, I wanted it removed. That same night, the diarrhea stopped and has not returned. Mrs. sent a note: "God bless you, for helping me with this terrible intestinal problem."

Case: Amy, age 32, toxic effect of a root canal.

Amy had exhausting headaches; she could barely get her husband off to work and two boys off to school before lying on the couch the rest of the day. Her physical exam and dental evaluations by her physician and dentist were normal. Amy's dentist told her she could possibly be pregnant, but this was not the case. Her next step was to see a chiropractor for her head pain.

The chiropractor was my son, Bruce, who pointed her in my direction to have her teeth checked. A full mouth x-ray and a CEDS exam revealed a toxic root canal treated tooth, the upper right second molar. Her previous dentist, who had done the root canal, said it was impossible for that tooth to be a problem. However, the removal of the root canal treated tooth stopped her headaches and her energy level returned to normal. Dr. Meinig, DDS, has established in his book *Root Canal Cover-Up Exposed!,* all root canal treated teeth are infected.

Dr. Boyd Haley has taught chemistry at the University of Kentucky for many years. He is also the founder of one of the leading toxicity testing labs in the world. His over one hundred references on the toxicity of root canals can be found on the IAOMT web site (www.iaomt.com). See Chapter 9. He estimates that about 25% of root canal treated teeth test out as "extremely toxic", and that another 50% of root canal treated teeth would be classified as "toxic". Root canal treated teeth become extremely toxic because once infected by anaerobic bacteria or by fungal infection, the body's immune system cannot fight off the infection. The body's immune system does not function in a dead tooth as there are no white blood cells present. The waste products from the treated root canal tooth can cause tooth abscesses, jawbone cavitations, and systemic health problems in the heart, the kidneys, the joints, the brain and elsewhere.

Case: Mrs. U., age 36, bonding materials affect health.

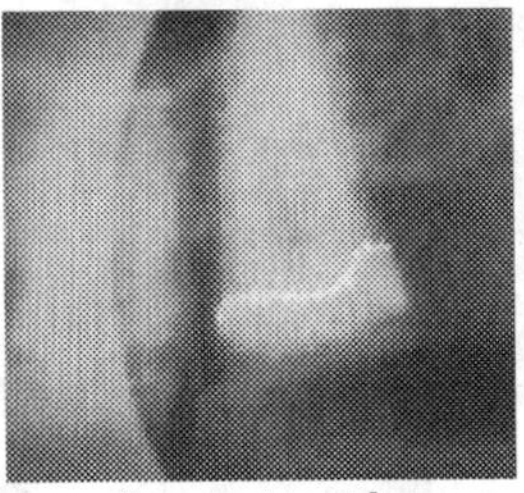

Mrs. U. noticed fatigue after a crown had been placed with a barium bonding material. Her x-ray confirmed a metal or metal oxide under her Premise Indirect (formally BelleGlass) crown (see bright white line under her crown), and CEDS supported my findings on the x-ray, which indicated that the barium in the bonding material was not compatible for her. After the old crown was removed and the new one was placed using Holistore, a compatible bonding material, Mrs. U. made a quick recovery from her fatigue.

Energy from dental materials has different effects on the health and the mental well being of patients. Remember, all dental materials must match the energy of the patient as closely as possible for good health. CEDS (a bio-feedback instrument) has proven many times to be a key factor in the selection of good restorative dental materials.

Case: Mr. Sam, 64, stomach pain.

Sam had stomach pain for ten years. A full mouth x-ray detected an infected first molar on the upper left side. Pain motivated Sam to see me for the removal of his tooth. His first statement when he returned for suture removal was "believe it or not, my stomach pain is gone."

Remember, upper first and second molars and lower first and

second bicuspids all influence the stomach, spleen and pancreas. Organs and tissue systems can be affected by: a root canal, (which is a dead tooth) decay, electric current from a filling, occlusion interference, metal fillings, toxic crowns, and dying or dead teeth.

After a filling is removed, CEDS evaluation aids us in telling if the tooth is vital (alive). Infections are not always visible at the end of the root. Without the CEDS evaluation it is very difficult to nearly impossible to find hidden infections in teeth. A vitality test using CEDS is more accurate, in most cases, than using an electric vitality tester.

Chapter 13

The Oral Cavity: A Cause of Health Problems

All the meridians from all the organ systems and teeth are connected to each other. Knowing these meridian energy connections makes it easier to understand the importance of the oral cavity. Health problems on one side of the oral cavity (right or left) can cross to the other side of the body causing sickness and pain problems. Body, mind and spirit are one and must be treated this way for good results.

Case: Nick, age 64, sore big toe related to lower first molar.

Nick's main complaint was pain in his left big toe causing him to limp. Nick's lower left first molar was extracted at age 15, but not until forty-nine years later did his big toe develop severe pain. After checking his lower first molar area with CEDS, I found an imbalance (infection). I surgically opened the gum tissue and jawbone, revealing a large cavitation (bone not yet healed) containing toxic dead bone tissue. Removal of this infected bone immediately stopped the pain in Nick's big toe. A major point in this case is the length of time between the cause and effect.

Everyone wants to know the cause and effect in minutes to hours. The health profession wants to relate specific symptoms to specific causes. For example, a patient walks into his medical doctor's office with a specific pain, wanting to know the cause. Health professionals need to be more open in recognizing that the oral cavity can be the cause of a wide variety of symptoms.

While reading the next case, use the Teeth and Body Energy chart to follow the relationship between teeth and organ systems.

Case: Mary Ann W., age 67, thirty years of extreme facial pain.

Mary Ann came to me in early September of 2005 with facial pain that passed over the right side of her face, and on to the top of her head. She was examined by thirty-three doctors from 1940 to 2005 for this pain. The only treatment she had received was pain medication.

Dr. Eleazar Kadile, M.D., in Green Bay, 60 miles from my office, advised Mary Ann to see me for a dental check up. He told her the teeth could be one of the main reasons for all of her problems from her toes to the top of her head. When she entered my office, her vibrations were those of a skeptic. I felt she was saying to herself, "another waste of time and money seeing my 34th doctor."

The first order of business was an oral exam, like she had had many times before by standard-of-care oral surgeons and dentists. Mary Ann told me the medical professionals had not looked in her mouth for the cause of her pain, neither had the dentists.

My evaluation went beyond standard care. This means looking at the entire body in relation to the oral cavity. Examining her mouth and her x-ray, I observed a combination of mixed metal fillings, resulting in galvanic current (electrical current from two or more different metals in the oral cavity). I found the following five problems in her mouth; 1) mercury silver amalgam fillings, 2) gold alloy fillings, 3) incompatible composite containing aluminum oxide, iron oxide, fluoride and/or barium, 4) root canals, and 5) a base metal bridge containing nickel. The upper right cuspid (eye tooth) and lateral tooth were root canals that had been placed at age 17. Checking her with CEDS, the root canals #6 and #7 led me to her main concern, head pain.

She said the pain had started soon after the root canals had been placed. Her upper #3 and #4 to #6 teeth (right side) held a nickel bridge. The Oral Potential Meter II recorded unacceptably high electrical activity in her bridge of 180 milli-volts, 6 micro-amps, and .56 micro-watts time seconds (energy) indicating possible decay and adding to her head pain. Refer to Chapter 3 Oral Potential Meter II Reveals Hidden Health Problems.

After receiving her permission, I used an easy technique to find the source of her pain. I placed a few drops of local anesthetic over the two root canals, and her pain stopped within a minute after the injection. Mary Ann's eyes filled with tears of joy at finding the cause. Injection of the anesthetic reduced the pain in her head and face like acupuncture, allowing her to go without pain medication until her appointment the following week.

Mary Ann returned for removal of #7 and #6, and I replaced the extracted root canals with a partial, and the nickel bridge #3 to #5 with a temporary bridge. Follow-up work included removal of all metals and metal oxide composites and placing non-metal fillings.

The patient's facial and head pain started again in 2008 when she allowed an endodontist to perform two more root canals, thinking it would save her teeth. I immediately canceled her head pain with local anesthetic to the two root canals #3 and #30. Mary Ann said, "This is the first relief of pain I have had all week". With the removal of her porcelain and nickel metal bridge #30 to #28, followed by removal of #30 and #3 root canal treated teeth, I stopped her pain.

The upper right lateral incisor tooth is related to the following organ and tissue systems: the rectum, anal canal, urinary bladder, frontal sinus, and sphenoid sinus. Joints affected by this tooth are: the posterior ankle, sacrococcygeal joint and posterior knee. The nose and the pineal gland are also related to this tooth. The upper cuspid tooth is related to the liver and gallbladder as well as to the back of the eye.

Case: Mr. Pete, 38, rectal bleeding.

Mr. Pete had rectal bleeding and itching for five years. A full mouth x-ray revealed the upper right central incisor tooth (tooth #8) had a root canal. Mr. Pete said the root canal had been done several years before his rectal trouble. Medication and ointments did not help the itching or the bleeding. I explained the relationship of the central incisor root canal to the rectum as a possible cause. He agreed to the removal and three days postoperatively, the itching and bleeding stopped.

Case: Mrs. Casey, age 52, sinus infection.

Mrs. Casey suffered with sinus problems for eight years. Her x-rays showed a root canal on the upper left central incisor #9. A large abscess (rotting infections next to the root of the tooth) could be seen on the x-ray, and at the end of the root. Removal of the central incisor tooth released green pus that flowed from the abscess. The next day she told me her sinus had drained the same green pus and this had fully opened her nasal airway. It had been years since she could breathe through her nose.

Case: Karen, age 28, low energy.

Karen's main complaints were low energy, dizziness, lack of concentration, and feeling faint. A full mouth x-ray showed two root canals on the upper two lateral incisors, with abscesses on both root tips. I replaced her fillings with non-metal oxide composites, and then extracted her root canals. Karen regained her energy, her dizziness disappeared, her concentration returned, and fainting was no longer a problem.

Remember: No tooth is worth losing a body function.

Chapter 14

Understanding Energy for Good Health

Computerized Electro-Dermal Screening (CEDS), a bio-feedback instrument is the fastest and most accurate way of finding compatible restorative materials for patients. I have checked many different dental materials and continue to look for ones my patients can live with. Finding a compatible restorative material is a key component in giving all patients better health.

Remember everything placed in the oral cavity has an energetic effect on the patient. A good example of hidden effect is a magnet with its ability to attract iron objects. A better example is a walk through security at the airport; a detector is able to tell if you are carrying metal. This same process happens when a filling is placed in a tooth. Your body energy-sensing field can pick up the energy from the metal or metal oxide fillings. Implant materials also need to be checked for compatibility on each patient.

The most consistent comment patients make after the metals are removed is, "I have more energy." I believe there are two reasons for this statement: first, removal of the electrical effects of the metals in the filling, and second, improvement in digestion and the immune system due to reduced toxicity. Controlled studies are needed to convince the professional health community of this effect.

Ann Summers, Ph.D. a research microbiologist showed that mercury produces antibiotic resistant bacteria in the intestinal tract; this alone is a good enough reason for not using mercury silver fillings. Most major health problems seem to begin in the gut from bad eating and drinking habits but they may also result from fungal infections due to mercury toxicity in the gut. This is the human factor. *You Are What You Ate*, by Sherry Rogers, M.D., and *Gut Psychology Syndrome*, by Natasha Campbell-McBride, M.D., are two books with great information on how the intestinal tract influences the mind and body.

Dentistry can make a difference. The following health histories demonstrate the dramatic changes occurring after compatible fillings are placed.

Case: Dr. O., M.D., age 41, anger.

Dr. O. came to me in 1995 after a long road of illness. He had resorted to doing natural things like caring for his own organic garden for food. He came to the conclusion that his mercury fillings were affecting him mentally and physically.

Anger, which he kept under control, was a major symptom of his illness. Removal of the mercury amalgams was his turning point, changing his anger into happiness. His health improved, he gained weight and has more energy, making him look and feel better than ever.

Case: Dr. S., M.D., age 66, eye sight.

Dr. S. came to me to have his metal fillings replaced. His eyesight improved with each filling he had removed. As the fillings were being removed, he said, "I can't believe I am seeing better already." From this time forward, due to his personal experience, Dr. S. began to see that dental problems, such as metal fillings and infection in the teeth and jaws, were affecting his patients' health. After his patients' fillings were replaced with compatible materials, and any infection in the teeth and jaws removed, his patients responded rapidly to his treatment.

As health professionals, we often see problems more clearly with our patient's health after we have corrected our own health. Throughout these chapters I have pointed out that the hazards and liabilities can be toxic metals, root canals, dead teeth, or infection in the jaws, many revealed with the use of CEDS that have been over looked with conventional exams.

Information for Dentists:

Dr. Voll, the father of electro acupuncture, found that all teeth are related to the eyes as well as to the 1st and 2nd vertebrae in the neck. They are also associated with other organ and tissue systems.

Case: Chuck, age 50, double vision.

While driving home from work, Chuck noticed that the signs did not look normal. He was experiencing double vision. The next day he went to his eye doctor who sent him to a specialist. This specialist placed a prism on his right eyeglass lens that allowed him to see one of everything. He was then scheduled to have his right eye muscle shortened to pull the right eye into alignment with his left eye. This meant the eye would be pulled from the socket to shorten a muscle.

My son, Bruce, Chuck's chiropractor, knew about the relationship of teeth to eyes and how it could be a major problem. Being a good friend of Chuck, Bruce advised him to have his teeth checked before eye surgery. Chuck came in the next day for a dental exam that included a full mouth x-ray and an Oral Potential Meter II electrical reading of each filling. Chuck's fillings registered the highest readings I had seen in 14 years. On the right side of his mouth he had mercury silver amalgam fillings, both on the upper and lower, that recorded double the electricity of the left side fillings. I told him I was not sure if the removal of the fillings would help his eyesight. Both Chuck and his wife agreed to have the mercury amalgams removed. My plan was to get rid of the electrical current (associated with decay) to see if this would bring the double vision back to normal with glasses.

At Chuck's next appointment, I worked on the right side of his mouth, removing all the mercury silver amalgam fillings. Removal was accomplished with low-speed drilling. To prevent Chuck from breathing toxic mercury vapor, I used The Clean Up Tip and the high vacuum suction at the chin. (Refer to chapter 4).

I discovered that between the teeth, at the bottom of the filling, tooth decalcification was taking place (a result of galvanic current), causing decay not seen on the x-ray. His insurance company evaluated the claim and paid for the replacement of his fillings. Dental literature points out that electrical current in the fillings will cause a loss of metal ions and of calcium from the tooth enamel, resulting in tooth decay. (Refer to Chapter 3).

Removal of the fillings on the right side allowed Chuck to remove the prism from his lens; he was able to see one of everything, except for his peripheral vision which still remained double. But at the next appointment, I removed the mercury silver amalgams from his upper and lower left side plus a root canal that was infected. The following day his eyesight was back to normal with glasses. NO EYE SURGERY! Dentistry does make a difference.

Case: Ron, Age 57, body pain.

Ron had pain in every joint, and needed a weekly shot of morphine just to have a few hours of comfort. His wife Joan, a registered nurse, cold- and hot-packed his painful joints to try and relieve any pain. She took Ron to every major medical clinic but found no cure for his pain. Pain medication was the only treatment. Dr. Wm. Faber, a physician at the Milwaukee Pain Clinic, referred Ron to me, thinking the mouth or teeth could be the cause of his pain. Ron's wife was very skeptical. She was sure I would just go on vacation with the money I would make from removing Ron's fillings. I put Ron through the standard procedures we do for new patients plus the Oral Potential Meter II, for an electrical check of his fillings.

Checking Ron's mouth, I found mixed metals, gold inlays, and crowns as well as mercury silver amalgam fillings; another case of mixed metals that resulted in the current known as oral galvanism. The Oral Potential Meter II readings were only slightly above normal, nothing that made me think that the electricity was the problem. However, research shows that the amount of current is not proportional to the severity of the health problems. Remember, every patient has his or her own level of sensitivity.

Removing Ron's three fillings on the upper left side, one gold inlay and two mercury amalgams was enough to stop the pain that night in one area of his body. Successful pain relief prompted him to continue having the fillings removed. After each appointment, on the way home (two hour drive), he would tell his wife where the pain had left his body. Ninety eight percent of Ron's pain was gone after the last metal filling had been removed.

Filling removal was completed in 1993 and, in 1996, he told me, "I have not mentioned this to anyone, but if you had not helped me, I would have committed suicide."

Ron's letter to the American Dental Association:

August 1, 1994

Ms. Pamela Clevenger
Senior Writer
Dept. of Public Info. & Ed.
American Dental Association
211 East Chicago Avenue
Chicago, IL 60611-2678

Dear Ms. Clevenger:

I am writing this letter in order to take exception to your response of June 15, 1994, to my wife's (Joan Seidl) letter regarding my health problems arising from mercury/silver amalgams and/or gold crowns.

Your statement regarding the U.S. Department of Health & Human Services' independent panel of experts (CCEHRP) stating "there is no scientific justification for refusing to have amalgam fillings or having them removed" is totally political rhetoric. The reason they say this is because they, (CCEHRP - U.S. Dept. of Health & Human Services - ADA) will not accept the countless documents from the people who have removed the metals from numerous patients and can see and document the improved health of these patients.

With regard to the ADA pamphlet *Facts About Dental Amalgam*, "mercury is used with other metals in dental amalgams and is safe". This statement is false. Mercury is a **POISON** and is considered a **HAZARDOUS MATERIAL**. Prior to putting the mercury amalgam into a person's tooth, it must be handled as a hazardous material and, according to EPA regulations, when it is removed it must be handled and disposed of as a hazardous material. If mercury is in a tooth, how can it then be considered **'SAFE'**?. This is political rhetoric!

Referring to a statement in the pamphlet "mercury is a naturally occurring element in the environment and some is always present in the human body", this is true. However, the statement in the pamphlet which reads "...the daily dosage of mercury released from dental amalgams is minuscule..." is political rhetoric. The USDA, U.S. Dept. of Health & Human Services and the EPA say we cannot consume too much fish or seafood from certain area waters because of high levels of mercury, yet mercury amalgams are placed in the body and release daily dosages. No one says how much mercury is released, yet it is **'SAFE'**? Again, political rhetoric!

With regard to the statement in the pamphlet of people being cured from illnesses when amalgam fillings are removed, it states the FDA and National Multiple Sclerosis Society have found no evidence and/or scientific evidence that disease, illness and

Ms. Pamela Clevenger
August 1, 1994
Page 2

general health conditions improve after removal of mercury/silver amalgams and/or gold. The reason they do not accept any documentation of improved health after amalgam removal is because no scientist can do a "scientific study" of the effects of amalgams using a control group and a placebo group.

The use of mercury/silver amalgams and gold in tooth restorations will produce electricity in the mouth. This electrical current will follow along the normal nerves in the human body in which a natural current is traveling from the nerve center to all areas of the body. This additional electricity being generated in the mouth is too much for the body to handle and, therefore, reacts in swelling of joints, pain and eventually deterioration of the healthy tissue. Also, mercury silver amalgams, after a period of years, expand and crack the tooth. These are the effects of metals in the teeth that I experienced.

The three doctors that I went to said: "I do not know what the problem is." One of the doctors, a specialist in rheumatology/arthritis, said: "I don't know, it could be arthritis, rheumatoid arthritis, or the start of multiple sclerosis", and also said that I may end up being a cripple. Does this last sentence sound familiar? Symptoms such as swelling of joints and fatigue closely resemble the symptoms of multiple sclerosis. A doctor not knowing what the illness is may diagnose multiple sclerosis when, in fact, the symptoms stem from mercury/silver amalgam fillings.

Everyday I thank God for the doctor that had experience diagnosing my symptoms and knew of doctors who could correct my problems. Today I'm a healthy 57 year old man doing 50-plus hours of physical work weekly and enjoying life tremendously, all because a great person removed the metals from my mouth.

Sincerely,

Ronald W. Seidl

Ronald W. Seidl

Case: Helen, age 64, ten years of sinus infection.

Helen's sinus drainage problem had lasted for ten years. Her major complaint was heavy sinus drainage that would not allow her to sing in church. Helen suspected her mercury fillings were the problem. I removed her three mercury amalgams at her request. Three days after removal and placement of non-metal fillings, her sinuses stopped draining. Helen's problem was solved and she could again sing in church.

Information for Dentists: Results of Metal Removal

As mentioned earlier, two things happen when metals are eliminated from the oral cavity, number one, electrical effects are eliminated, and number two, the immune system and digestion improve for better health.

In the article reprinted in Chapter 8, Dr. Eggleston states that a patient's immune system can double after the removal of metal fillings. There are eighty one references to metals at the end of Dr. Eggleston's article. In chapter 5, Dr. Harold Kristal's study also shows how metals depress the immune system.

Case: Matt, age 34, memory loss.

Matt, a student at the University of Upper Michigan, was finishing his Doctorate degree in physics. His mother called me from Virginia Beach about seeing him because he had lost his ability to calculate out two matrixes in his head at the same time and come up with the right answer. Figuring out math problems had now became impossible. Matt's Ph.D. exam was coming up in three weeks. Removing Matt's metal fillings brought back his mental functions, and he received the highest grade on the Ph.D. exam in the United States.

Case: Edward, age 58, memory loss.

Edward, an engineer from Minneapolis, MN, had the same memory loss symptoms as Matt. He came to see me because he could no longer add large numbers. Losing his ability to add caused this engineer to worry about losing his job. After removal of all of his metal fillings, his mathematical skills returned.

Case: June, age 53, constipation.

June suffered with constipation for nine long years. Her oral exam revealed one mercury amalgam filling on the side of the lower right second molar. Remember that lower molars are related to the function of the large intestine and lung.

After removing the mercury silver amalgam from her molar I replaced it with a compatible composite. She returned in eight weeks, excited and smiling. She said, "You will never guess what you have done for me. My nine years of constipation are gone!"

The effects of electricity from the filling could have had an influence on her constipation. Removal of a mercury silver amalgam had allowed her bowel to once again function normally. Constipation can be a symptom of low thyroid function, and low thyroid function is a common effect of both mercury and fluoride. Hypothyroidism may afflict as many as 12% of the adult females in the United States.

Case: Dan, age 74, breathing problem.

Dan, a World War II dental technician, had shortness of breath, muscle cramps in his legs, and brain fog. His oral exam revealed four mercury silver amalgams. He wanted the fillings removed to see if his health would improve.

I used a vacuum at his chin and a Clean Up Tip over the filling to capture the mercury fumes. Without the high suction vacuum and clean-up tip, Dan, as well as my assistant and I, would have inhaled the dangerous toxic mercury fumes. On Dan's return appointment he had a big smile while telling about the change in his breathing when walking. "No more problem sinuses, my lungs opened up, I can breathe again without effort."

Case: Doug, age 32, lost sense of balance.

Doug, a world-class mountain climber, has climbed in Tibet, South America, Alaska, and in the United States. Doug came to me on a referral from Dr. Stone because he lost his sense of balance, which ended his mountain climbing career. I removed all of his metal fillings, replacing them with a non-metal filling material and his balance returned. Doug continued climbing with his friends.

Case: Leona, age 65, cough of 20 years duration.

Leona coughed for twenty years, sometimes so severely, she felt like she would pass out. Examinations by three Ear, Nose and Throat specialists could not find any reason for this symptom.

I checked her one mercury filling with the Oral Potential Meter II, which recorded a very high electrical reading. Her lower metal partial added to her persistent cough, an electrical-related problem. I removed the mercury silver amalgam filling, replacing it with a compatible composite. I asked Leona to leave her metal partial out of her mouth and, by the very next day, the cough was gone. Removal of metals in her mouth stopped her persistent cough.

Case: Linda, age 28, collapsed on the floor.

Linda came to me in 1992 for a dental evaluation. Before Linda's problem arose, she had placed first or second in the cross country skiing event, part of the Badger Games held in Wisconsin every winter. One day Linda fell to the floor. She made her way to the phone and called for help. Years of tests and exams failed to provide a reason for her collapse. Linda researched the library looking for answers, but none were found to help her condition.

One day her mother called and asked if she had considered her teeth as a cause of her problem. This suggestion brought

Linda to my office where a full mouth x-ray showed a number of fillings and a root canal in the lower left second bicuspid, along with a mercury amalgam filling in the bone at the gum line.

All metal fillings had to be replaced along with the extraction of the root canal. I also removed the mercury filling in her jaw on the backside of the root canal. Removing the metals helped her feel better; however the turning point was the removal of the root canal, which allowed Linda to regain her former level of health.

Chapter 15

Taking Responsibility for Your Health

Compare a dentist who knows only how to fill a tooth, to a dentist who uses CEDS, to find the best restorative material for your energy. A dentist using CEDS is able to tell you if the tooth is healthy or infected, and whether or not the jaw is free of infection. Dr. Voll's Teeth and Body Energy chart will show you which organ systems are influenced by each tooth, and CEDS can help the dentist make the decisions that can lead to a good end result.

Read *The High Blood Pressure Hoax*, by Sherry Rogers, M.D. In this book, Dr. Rogers explains why it is important to educate yourself about minerals and the vascular system. She stresses that you must take care of yourself when your doctor is not doing the job.

Balanced readings with the CEDS instrument need to be in the 50 to 60 range and holding solid. Instrument sound should be even with no change in the tone; this even tone indicates a balanced energy condition.

Imbalanced readings are indicated with a high or very low reading followed by a tone change starting with a higher tone and falling to a lower tone. Remember, the instrument does not actually diagnose anything. Diagnosis is done by the health care professional, as is the treatment.

My method of checking teeth with CEDS is to first remove all the filling material from the teeth. Each tooth has to have a balanced reading using the (Lymph 2) point for the upper and lower jaw. This point will indicate if there is infection in the teeth or the jaws. A high reading and a drop in tone tells the health care professional that a dead tooth or infection in the jaws is present.

Patients will ask questions about the readings and what they mean, and they quickly learn the difference between good readings and problem readings. Surprisingly, many patients pick up on the change in sound the CEDS makes when the jaws and teeth are being tested. Remember, the more informed patients are, the better the questions they can ask. Knowledge is power, for both the dentist and the patient.

Using the most compatible filling material is vitally important to the health of the tooth and the patient. Before testing, remove any metal from the patient's body, including jewelry or electronics such as watches, car key openers, and hearing aids, as these can affect the energy in the oral cavity. Other energy interference can come from: labels in clothing, underwire in bras, hair dye, cosmetics containing petroleum and cadmium, synthetic clothing, perfume, after-shave cologne, and fluoride in any form (toothpaste, sealants for teeth, or treatments for children's teeth). These all have a disruptive effect. Silk, linen, cotton, wool, and clothing without moth and fire retardant, are the best choices for good health.

Electromagnetic frequencies from just about every electrical device and even wall outlets can affect sensitive patients. Go to www.stetzerelectronic.com to get more information on this problem.

When a balanced reading cannot be found, consider irradiated food or water heated in a microwave and/or pesticides as the hidden cause. CEDS is undoubtedly one of the easiest and fastest methods for finding many hidden health problems. It is true that not all patients have the same sensitivities. However there is a consistent pattern: a high percent of the time, sickness is related to the above listed items along with interferences from the oral cavity.

Long standing health problems are a clue that the oral cavity needs to be checked using every method available. Recall this good example; May Ann, age 68, had facial pain for thirty years, with the cause literally right under her nose. Root canals on the upper right lateral incisor and cuspid directly affected her facial and head pain. Think of the money she could have saved in travel, tests, examinations and prescriptions, not to mention the pain, had her dentist or physician been aware of this connection.

Important For the Dentist:

A good starting point for health professionals, along with learning CEDS, is study of the Teeth and Body Energy chart. Dentists, because of their special knowledge of the oral cavity, are able to improve their patients' health when other methods have failed. A close examination of x-rays, will show toxic metal fillings as well as metal oxide composites. Remember most composites contain aluminum oxide, iron oxide, fluoride and/or barium. Fluoride (a neurotoxin), found in most composites, cannot be seen on x-ray, but is easily detected with CEDS. Dentists are greatly aided by knowing the tooth-to-organ relationships when reading patient medical histories.

Patients' medical histories are a major clue to finding an organ influenced by an infected tooth or jaw. My German teachers said third molars (wisdom teeth) are always associated with body and heart problems. Pathology in the jaws and wisdom teeth areas are found with CEDS, and after surgery, cavitations can be checked with CEDS to be as sure as possible that the jaw bone is clean and free of pathology (infection).

Dentists skilled in the use of CEDS have eliminated hundreds of cavitations, adding to their patients' health. A study of the heart to wisdom teeth link is very difficult because of the lack of communication between the two professions that could connect the oral cavity to the patient's overall health. Most medical doctors believe care of the oral cavity belongs only to the dentist and that body care belongs only to the medical doctor. WRONG! Health professionals have to work together for the good of the patient.

Chapter 16

Detoxification

Once a patient has all dental amalgam fillings and other toxic metals removed from the oral cavity it should become much easier to remove the mercury and other toxins that have been stored in the body's tissues. A major purpose of amalgam removal is to allow the body to move into this vigorous detoxification ("detox") phase. It is as though the body gives up on trying to detoxify itself as long as it is being subjected every day to the mercury released from the amalgam fillings.

But there can be other barriers to detoxification that can prevent the body from moving into the detox phase. These barriers include an overly acidic body pH, mineral and vitamin deficiencies, the presence of infections, poor circulation, and problems with the organs of elimination – the kidneys, the liver and the bowel. For sicker patients, an evaluation by a health care practitioner other than the dentist before amalgam replacement can help identify the existence of any problem areas. These should be addressed, if possible, prior to amalgam replacement. By resolving constipation, for example, and improving the function of the kidneys, liver and gut, the process of removing amalgam fillings by a qualified dentist becomes even safer and smoother.

The mercury toxic patient is usually low in such vital nutrients as magnesium, zinc, vitamin C and the B vitamins. This is because these important nutrients get used up in the never-ending fight to protect the body against mercury's attacks, and by supplementing with the needed minerals and vitamins early on, prior to amalgam removal, the patient will feel better, and experience a safer amalgam removal and more successful detoxification. Also, when the body has plenty of essential minerals, it is more willing to let go of toxic elements.

Sea salt, which contains a broad range of essential minerals, is important to use, rather than table salt (sodium chloride) which is best avoided. One fourth teaspoon of sea salt should be added to each quart of water that is drunk, in order to have proper hydration from the water. The kidneys are helped by drinking plenty of water every day.

Liver function can be assisted in a number of ways. An excellent supplement is silymarin, which is naturally derived from the milk thistle seed. The liver is an important digestive organ, since it secretes bile, which is needed to emulsify and help digest fats. The liver stores bile in the gall bladder and, when fats come down into the small intestines for digestion, the gall bladder squeezes out the bile that is needed for digestion. But if the person is detoxifying, something else is coming along in the bile: mercury or other toxic metals. They are being dumped into the intestines to be carrying into the bowel and eliminated in a bowel movement. The liver has cleaned the mercury and other heavy metals out of the blood that it filters. So, to allow the body to get rid of the toxins that have been sent by the liver into the bile, the body needs a reasonably good bowel function.

"Transit time" is the time that food takes to pass through the GI tract and exit the body at the other end. For detox supplements to work effectively, the transit time should be under twenty hours. Slow transit time and constipation are often a problem for the toxic patient, because mercury, fluoride and other toxins tend to cause low thyroid function ("hypothyroidism"). This low thyroid function tends produce fatigue, low energy, inactivity and a sluggish bowel. The patient may be able to speed up transit time by eating more high-fiber natural foods, and drinking more water. Colon therapy and other forms of professional help may be needed to improve bowel function and clear up constipation.

Infections such as Lyme disease are all too common and can go undiagnosed for years. Lyme and mercury poisoning work synergistically, each making the other one harder to deal with. Fungal infections are another bane of mercury-poisoned patients. Mercury tends to promote the development of the fungal form of the common yeast, Candida albicans. Other common causes of fungal yeast overgrowth are antibiotics, especially when they are used heavily and for a long period of time. While Candida albicans is present in any healthy person, this normally harmless yeast can organize itself into a parasitical, aggressive fungal colony which can attach to intestinal walls and punch holes there, allowing the passage of undigested foods into the body. This "leaky gut syndrome" is associated with most food sensitivities. The parasitic Candida colonies can cause intestinal bloating and indigestion, vaginal yeast infections, esophageal reflux, sinus problems, arthritic symptoms, brain fog, food cravings and much more.

The answer to these difficult and painful problems is to follow a carefully restricted anti-fungal diet (no sugar, no sweets!), use anti-fungal supplements such as monolaurin and lactoferrin, and take special supplements to help the gut heal. But safe amalgam removal and a safe, natural detox is fundamental to the success of any anti-fungal program. Too often, doctors attack the fungal problem head-on with heavy use of anti-fungal drugs, while ignoring the need to alter the patient's diet, remove amalgams, and detoxify their body. Such a short-sighted approach just doesn't work, long term.

What should ***not*** occur before amalgam removal is aggressive detox. The use of powerful drugs such as DMPS or DMSA, prior to amalgam removal, often aggravates the patient's symptoms. Even post-amalgam removal, the drugs seem to be the riskiest way to detoxify, as they produce a high rate of toxic side effects and should be used with great caution, if at all. Because safer, more effective supplements are now available, the use of aggressive detox drugs can be avoided altogether.

The non-drug choices fall roughly into the following categories: helpful foods, helpful exercises, massage therapy, skin methods, and oral supplements. Leading the list of foods that aid in detoxification are eggs, garlic and onions, which provide sulfur, selenium and other helpful nutrients. At the same time, sugar, alcohol and caffeine are to be avoided, as they make the body chemistry too acidic. Most toxic people have a body pH which is too acidic and should adjust their diets to include alkaline-forming foods that help shift the chemistry back to a slightly alkaline state.

Exercise, like diet, should be carefully tailored to the needs and abilities of the individual patient. Avoid over-doing it and causing injury. Gentle exercise such as walking, biking, or bouncing on a rebounder, if kept within the abilities of the patient, can help get the lymphatic fluids moving. The lymphatic fluids carry toxins out of the body's tissues and into the blood where they can then be removed by the liver and the kidneys. Massage is especially important for the patient who is unable to be physically active.

One or more "skin methods" are normally a helpful part of any detox program. The skin is an organ of detoxification and sweating is an effective way of getting rid of toxic wastes, as long as the sweat is showered off before it can be re-absorbed. If kidney or liver function is impaired, the body will rely on the skin to an even greater degree to rid itself of toxins, and rashes and/or dark pimples on the skin may appear as obvious signs that the skin detox is happening. Some of the traditional skin methods are the warm bath, perhaps with baking soda and/or Epsom salts added to the water. A warm bath with bathing clays is excellent. A Far Infrared sauna and steam sauna followed by a shower to get rid of the sweat is also good and is a detox method that is centuries old in many cultures. The skin methods vary in price, but some of the simpler methods, such as skin brushing, are very affordable and should be performed daily.

Most patients choose one aggressive oral supplement to complement a well chosen diet, and use several different skin methods, alternating them from day to day.

Supplements

There are dozens of oral supplements for the more aggressive detox. Ads for these detox products can be found in the DAMS newsletter and in most natural health magazines. Every year new oral supplements are placed on the market, adding to the rapidly-growing industry of detoxification products.

The most notable entry into the detox market, introduced in the summer of 2008 is OSR, (Oxidative Stress Relief). Its developer, Dr. Boyd Haley, is widely admired because he has tirelessly spoken out on the health hazards of mercury and the need to ban it in dentistry and medicine. OSR is classified as a food supplement and not a drug; it makes no claims to treat, prevent or cure any disease or illness. But it is an excellent anti-oxidant that has been shown to boost the body's level of glutathione, an important natural detoxifier of mercury and other toxic metals, and is able to scavenge dangerous free radicals, such as the hydroxyl radical.

Prior to its being marketed, OSR was extensively tested on animals and was found to be very safe and non-toxic. Unlike drugs such as DMPS or DMSA, OSR does not deplete the body of zinc or other essential trace minerals. Use in humans has also shown that OSR is safe and beneficial. OSR is currently being marketed to physicians and other health care professionals, but not directly to the consumer. Healthcare professionals may order OSR by e-mailing the company CTI Science at behaley@ctiscience.com. Will OSR become a new leader in the field of detox supplements? It is still very new and more time is needed to allow us to evaluate its clinical value.

Resources: DAMS Information Guide and the DAMS Newsletter, Dental Truth, which is published several times a year. As the months and years go by, these DAMS resources will track what is new in detox methods and products and how well they work. Call 800-311-6265 from the US or Canada, or e-mail DAMS at dams@usfamily.net.

Chapter 17

Dental Materials Are One of the Keys to Health

Compatible dental materials are a major key to good health, since dental materials need to match the patient's body energy. Product developers of composites, dental gold, plastics and base metals have little knowledge of the energetic effect these dental materials have on a patient's health. I use CEDS on all patients to test for sensitivity to a particular dental material, thereby avoiding a negative reaction.

Of the following dental materials, the first three are consistently compatible, and I am presently using them. However, the fourth and fifth materials need to be tested with CEDS on each patient for compatibility.

(1)Holistore by Den-Mat is the most compatible composite. It contains no aluminum oxide, iron oxide, or barium oxide, making it a very compatible metal oxide free filling as well as containing no fluoride. It is not opaque on an x-ray, therefore it looks like decay. Holistore is used in low stress chewing areas such as on the side of the tooth at the gingival or gum line, and on the chewing surface of the tooth if the cavity is small. Because the filling material is not as hard as enamel, Holistore fillings need to be checked every six months to be either resurfaced or replaced if wear is noticed. Holistore Light, a less viscous version of Holistore, is used to bond Premise Indirect (formally BelleGlass) inlays, onlays, crowns, and bridges onto the prepared teeth. Only the more viscous (thicker) version of Holistore, mentioned above, is used for small fillings. Thank you to Den-Mat Corporation for making Holistore. Den-Mat is one of the very few companies that listen to the dentists and fill their requests. To purchase Holistore call Den-Mat Corporation phone: 800 - 433-6628 extension 6222, ask for knowledgeable sales person.

(2) For the common case of larger cavities and cavities on major chewing surfaces, a Holistore filling will not work. I would then use an inlay made out of another very biocompatible material, Premise Indirect (formally BelleGlass) unshaded. This unshaded Premise Indirect is 80% glass and 20% resin binder, and is processed at a dental lab. Its hardness is close to that of enamel; no shading is recommended for crowns, inlays, and short span bridges. Shading contains iron oxide to make a crown or bridge look like a natural tooth. In most cases, energy from the iron oxide is not compatible with the patient's health. Various adverse symptoms can be associated with the effects of iron oxide shading in the bonded restorations.

(3) A mixture of cadmium-free plastic, Vitalon 1060, manufactured by Fricke (see appendix) International is used for partials and dentures. Hardening of this plastic powder and liquid mixture is done in a water bath for twenty hours and cured at one hundred and sixty-seven degrees Fahrenheit. A long curing time of the plastic dentures or partials removes the liquid (monomer) making the plastic more compatible.

(4) Point 4, a composite filling manufactured by Kerr Company, has good wear strength, ease of application, and polishes to a smooth finish. Point 4 does contain barium, so CEDS must be used to check each patient for compatibility with this material.

(5) Bistite II DC is a bonding agent for crowns, inlays and bridges manufactured by Tokuyama. It does contain some aluminum oxide, so CEDS must be used to check each patient for compatibility with this material.

Most of my patients who have done their homework request a CEDS evaluation of dental restorative materials for compatibility as well as for checking for infection in their teeth and jaws.

Temporary materials are not tolerated over a long period. They are used for a week or two to protect the tooth while the permanent restoration is being made. Protemp 3 Garant by 3M is one of the best and most accurate temporary materials I am currently using. All dental materials should be tested with CEDS, on patients' lymph, nervous, circulation, and endocrine conductance points for compatibility.

A simple way to check composite filling materials is to x-ray them on a flat surface. If the material shows up on the x-ray you know it contains a metal oxide. Then check the material with CEDS on the patient.

This x-ray shows the crown was placed using barium containing bonding material. Barium is in the bright white line under the crown.

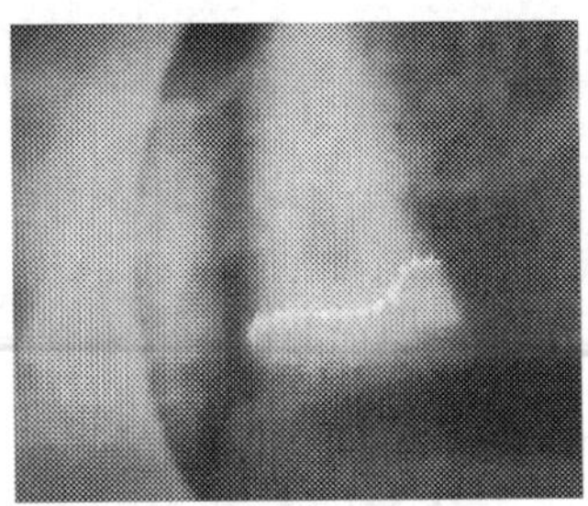

There is a composite that is free of barium oxide, and does not show on x-ray; however it does contain fluoride, making it unacceptable. Fluoride in composites can only be detected with CEDS or you can read the MSDS (Material Safety Data Sheet) for the material. All restorative materials are required to have an MSDS on their content. MSDS sheets are made available at your request through your dental office. My dental salesperson said if the fluoride is below a certain percentage, the manufacture does not have to list it on the MSD Sheet. Any amount of fluoride is toxic.

A true test of the restorative material is how the patient reacts. Listen to your patients, they will tell you if they notice any abnormal changes, such as increased heart rate, disturbances in sleeping patterns, shortness of breath, mental fog, joint pain, or digestive problems and more.

Be aware that adverse reactions to some of these dental materials can occur within seconds, while other reactions take weeks or months. Use your CEDS to choose the best restorative material. It can save time and money for the patient, and the dentist can avoid having to replace incompatible fillings.

Many dentists prefer using gold for restorations because of its lasting qualities. However, the body's cells must make an adjustment to any filling material, even gold. Many patients tell me their health made a change for the better after having non-metal fillings placed. Patients who are having their fillings removed for health reasons are not concerned with looks (aesthetics); they want good health. In other words, these patients are sick of being sick. Most health care professionals outside of dentistry check everything with standard procedures, but fail to look at the teeth and jaws. Standard physical exams need to include checking fillings for electrical current, for incompatible dental materials and for toxic infected jawbone areas or teeth (including root canal treated teeth). At the Paracelsus Clinic in Switzerland, Dr. Thomas Rau requires all root canals to be removed either prior to, or on arrival for medical treatment.

Dentists must be alert for a patient's adverse reaction to dental materials. For example, fumes from the removal of restorations that are toxic, such as mercury silver amalgams, toxic gold alloys and base metal alloys that contain nickel and other toxic materials. Care must be taken with the patient when removing any restorations!

Case: Mr. T., age 48, brain fog

I removed the upper and lower mercury amalgams on the right side for Mr. T. and three days later he called to tell me how sick he was after the removal. He was dizzy, his stomach was upset, and he suffered brain fog.

Mr. T.'s background is in metallurgy, and he knew that mercury fumes from the mercury silver fillings were responsible for his sick feeling. On his second appointment, to remove the remaining mercury fillings, he suggested we use a household vacuum cleaner placed in the hall with the hose held to his chin, which pulled the mercury fumes away from his face. These fumes can be avoided with the proper vacuum systems. He called the next day, to report he was feeling good and having none of the previous symptoms.

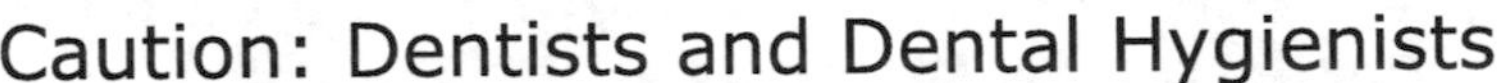

Caution: Dentists and Dental Hygienists

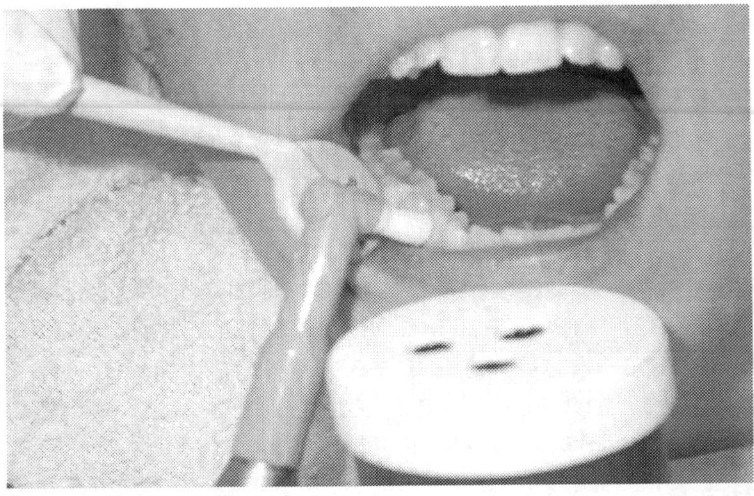

A separate vacuum must be used to remove the toxic mercury fumes while drilling or polishing teeth with silver mercury amalgam fillings. Advise the patient to hold the vacuum hose firmly to the chin with the mouth open; mercury fumes are emitted for approximately two minutes.

All patients should follow a detoxification program after having their teeth cleaned and after removal of mercury amalgam fillings. Information on metal detoxification can be found in the books *Detoxify or Die*, and *High Blood Pressure Hoax*, by Sherry Rogers, M.D. Call DAMS, 800-311-6265' for more information about safe detox options.

The oral cavity is one of the main sources of hidden health problems. The following cases are outstanding examples of degeneration from root canals, cavitations, or dying teeth. Many times these infections cannot be found on x-ray but are easily detected with CEDS.

Case: Dr. Cook, age 60, painful elbow.

I had a painful elbow that came from an infected tooth. The elbow became so painful; I felt I would have to quit dentistry. While attending a seminar on computerized electro-dermal screening, our instructor found my upper right first bicuspid (tooth #5) to be infected. When the tooth was checked with conventional methods, all appeared normal

Fortunately, CEDS found the cause of the problem. I had to make a choice! My choices were to either have the tooth removed, or have a root canal done. Dr. Bill Barton, a dentist in Green Bay, consented to pull the tooth, although he did have second thoughts about removing such a normal looking tooth, as viewed on x-ray.

Dr. Barton surgically removed the tooth by making an incision through the gum tissue, to expose the bone. Using a drill, he removed the bone over the root to allow the tooth to come out without using excessive pressure.

A first bicuspid has two roots that are, in many cases, very likely to break when the tooth is pulled. In this case both root tips broke off and had to be surgically removed. The cheek side root tip came out looking perfect. Immediately I said, "I just had a good tooth pulled!" Next, Dr. Barton took out a small amount of bone to remove the inside root. When it was taken out, there, on the tip of the root, was a small abscess. It was clear that the infected tooth had been the cause of my painful elbow.

Yet, I wonder why this tooth went bad and caused a systemic health issue that almost forced me to give up dentistry? The answer was found when I broke the tooth open looking for a clue to the cause of the death of my tooth. I broke the tooth in half, but luck was really with me; the break was exactly where the crown and root came together. I had expected to see two open root canals; but one canal was open and the other root canal was calcified shut. Blood, nerve and lymph supply were all cut off, allowing an abscess to form at the end of this root.

The body does not like dead tissue and tries to get rid of it at any cost. My elbow pain directed me to the cause by following the large intestine meridian. Remember, the large intestine meridian passes through the elbow and through this infected tooth #5. Within ten minutes after my tooth removal I knew the elbow was on its way to feeling better and the pain was dramatically reduced. Complete recovery took three full months. This case points out why all health professionals need to have a working knowledge of the oral cavity and the meridians associated with the different teeth and organs. It also confirms Dr. Voll's principle that the oral cavity plays an important role in total health.

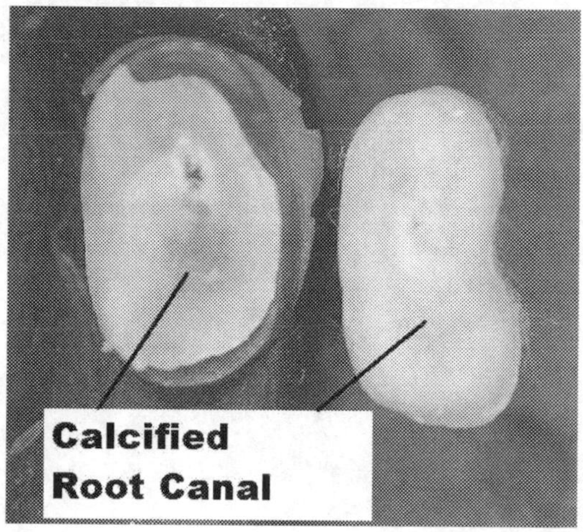

Photo of my tooth separated; on the left is the crown and on the right is the root, with the one root canal calcified shut.

Important Point for Dentists

Anything on a meridian (energy line of force in the body) can cause a problem on that meridian. The meridian associated with my dead tooth is related to the large intestine (find tooth #5 on tooth-energy chart, appendix B). You may refer to Dr. Speckhart's book: *An Electrodermal Analysis of Biological Conductance,* page 86, for a picture of the large intestine meridian.

The path of the large intestine meridian is as follows: a line of energy goes from the first finger up the arm past the wrist to the elbow (my pain area), over the front of the shoulder, up the neck to the jaw passing over the first and second molar on the lower jaw. It then passes to the upper jaw crossing the first and second bicuspids and ending at the edge of the nose.

Having a painful elbow and losing a tooth was an eye-opening lesson. I give my appreciation to Dr. Andrew Landerman for his skill in finding my infected tooth and to Dr. Bill Barton for the removal of the tooth. What would have been the medical treatment for my painful elbow, if I hadn't use CEDS to find the true cause? Injections of a steroid for the rest of my life or waiting until the tooth would become painful? It makes one think of what may be causing any discomfort. Dentists do make a difference!

Chapter 18

X-rays

How good are X-rays for finding infection?

Understand that the outer layer of jawbone is next to the cheek, and the inner layer of jawbone is alongside the tongue. Clarity of the tooth on an x-ray depends on the thickness of these two layers of bone; this is a major reason why infections are hidden on an x-ray. Dentists may refuse to remove a tooth when they cannot see an infected area at the end of the root. Infection is often hidden behind, or between, the roots, where it cannot be seen on an x-ray.

My tooth loss was a result of a nerve canal being calcified shut, causing its death. Symptoms are not always in the mouth! In my case, a painful elbow forced me to find the cause; standard medical protocols would have likely treated it differently.

It is critical for health professionals to know the basic path of the acupuncture meridians with regard to the teeth and organ tissue systems. With this knowledge, in many cases they can save patients pain, time, and money.

Look carefully at the picture and the x-ray of Margo's teeth, my next case.

Case: Margo, age 35, pulp stone.

A pulp stone is calcification inside the pulp chamber of the tooth; it slowly strangles the nerve and blood supply. Pulp stones are unusual; however we must consider them as a cause of pathology in the tooth.

Margo's case started with an infected root canal on the upper second bicuspid. This second bicuspid was extracted and a bridge was bonded to the first bicuspid and first molar to replace this tooth. Within a year the first molar died from the pulp stone cutting off its blood supply. In the x-ray on the right, see the large pulp stones in both the first and the second molar. The picture on the left shows the pulp stone in the extracted 1st molar.

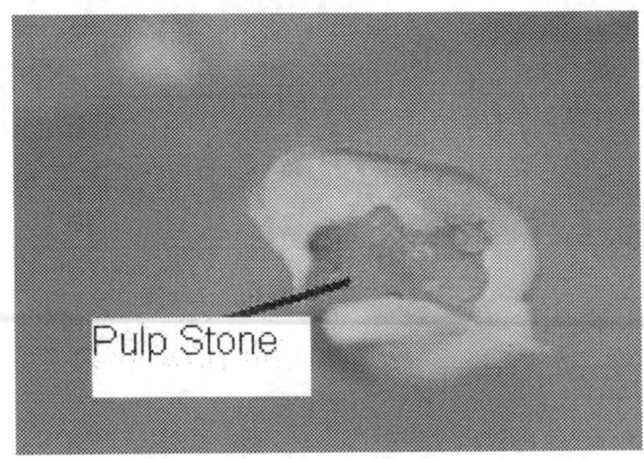

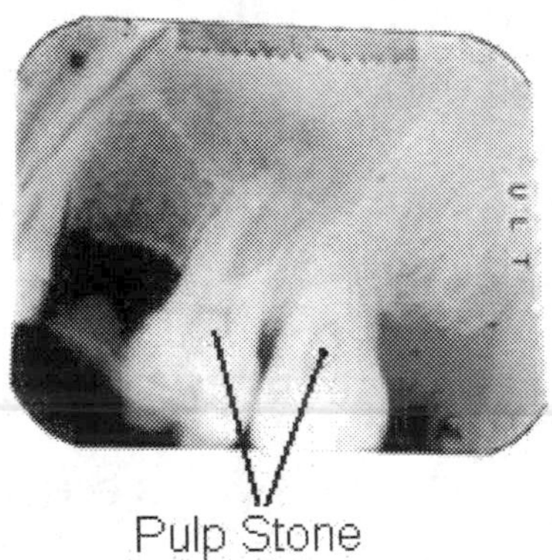

Information for the Dentist

More than any other health care professional, dentists are in the best position to help patients with health problems related to the oral cavity. Dentists will be first care providers in the near future. With their understanding of the Teeth and Body chart, dentists can rule out the oral cavity as the cause for unknown symptoms.

Remember the case of Nick's big toe? Nick's painful big toe was caused by an infection in the jaw, where forty-five years earlier a lower left first molar had been pulled. The problem was solved when CEDS found the infection. Removing this infection immediately stopped the toe pain. Symptoms are not always an immediate effect; the cause and the resulting symptom can be from minutes apart to even years apart.

Patients may exhibit a variety of symptoms, all arising from the same problem in the oral cavity. Here are some good examples of toxic causes that produce varied effects: mercury silver amalgams, dental gold restorations, metal appliances to replace teeth, toxic plastics for dentures, and infection in teeth and in the jawbone.

As more patients demand CEDS testing, this procedure will find its way into all dental and medical schools, stimulating a deeper awareness of the association of the oral cavity with sickness and pain.

Chapter 19

Finding a Suitable Holistic Dentist

A holistic dentist considers the patient's health from the time they walk into the office until their dental health is improved, through placing compatible fillings, removing infected teeth, clearing up infections in the jaw, detoxifying heavy metals and nutritional support.

When screening and interviewing holistic dental offices what should we look for? Ideally holistic dental offices should be free of perfume, cologne, and dental medication odors, have natural fiber carpets or hardwood floors throughout the office, be located a safe distance from high power lines, have no toxic developer solutions for x-rays, and have two high vacuum systems available for mercury fume removal. Remember to ask questions and expect the answers best for your health.

The first question to ask the dentist is, "Have you considered that health problems could be linked to the mouth?"

My advice is to study and understand how metal fillings can be a danger to health. If the dentist does not know that metals and metal oxides can be toxic, seek another dentist.

CEDS can be used to check all dental materials for your health. Some patients can tolerate metal and metal oxide fillings for a long time. But very few dentists understand the effects of toxic metal oxides in composites. It is crucial to know that composites that contain aluminum oxide, iron oxide, fluoride or barium, are a burden to your entire mental and physical health.

Every patient needs to be checked for his/her tolerance for barium in composites using the CEDS unit. Patients can learn more about toxic metals on the internet by typing in: metal toxicology.

The following materials are used in dentistry: gold, alloys, platinum, titanium, cadmium, mercury silver amalgams, aluminum oxide, iron oxide, fluoride, stainless steel or a silver-like metal containing a nickel alloy metal. All these metals have a negative energetic effect on our health. Be aware that the immune system is impaired by having metal fillings. See chapter 8, information by Dr. Eggleston and chapter 5, information by Dr. Harold Kristal.

Three ways for checking filling materials:

1. Ask for a Material Safety Data sheets, (MSDS). All restorative fillings have a MSDS telling the contents of the dental materials. If the description has any of the above materials, it should be a red flag.

2. Have an x-ray taken of the dental material the dentist wants to use. If the dental material shows up on the x-ray it contains a metal or metal oxide, another red flag.

3. Find a dentist who is skilled in using CEDS for finding compatible restorative dental materials or the restorative filling materials mentioned in this book. All health professionals have access to this information, but it does take time to learn and develop the skill to use CEDS. Look for a dentist who will consider your health first.

CEDS helps find the balance between the energy in the filling material and your own energy field. The bottom line is how well you do with the filling material after it is placed. Few health professionals have any idea of the reaction patients can have from fillings, root canals, dead teeth, or from the toxic affect from infection in the jaws (cavitations). Again, remember all root canals are infected!

For more information, visit International Academy of Oral Medicine and Toxicology web site www.iaomt.com ; Price Pottenger Foundation, and George Meinig's book, *The Root Canal Cover Up Exposed!*

Ask the dentist if he or she uses low speed for all drilling.

High-speed drilling can kill teeth by pulling projections in the dentinal tubules out of the dentine. Open dentinal tubules allow bacteria to pass into the pulp killing the tooth. Low speed drilling is safer and kinder to the tooth. Preparing the tooth for a new filling, crown or inlay with low speed drilling will save many teeth.

High speed drilling runs at 350,000 revolutions per minute which is one of the main reasons for tooth sensitivity and dead teeth. High speed drilling raises the temperature of the tooth, at the point of drilling, by 12 degrees centigrade. Water and air on the drill, at the point of contact, cannot cool the tooth adequately.

Low speed drilling runs at 20,000 revolutions per minute; this is the speed recommended for removing metal restorations and for preparing teeth for fillings. See Dr. Turk's article: "Iatrogenic Damage from High Speed Drilling", in Chapter 4.

Patient: "Do you check each tooth with CEDS after all the filling is removed, and do you also check with CEDS for infection in the jaws where teeth have been extracted or are missing?"

Dentist: "I remove all of the filling material in each tooth and check the tooth with CEDS for vitality. Next, I restore these good teeth followed by a CEDS evaluation of any infection in the jaws. Your health and health of your mouth will depend on these steps for compatible fillings."

All wisdom teeth extraction sites need to be checked with CEDS. Wisdom teeth areas are cross checked against their related organ systems (heart and small intestine). Checking all the missing teeth areas on the first visit is important for the patient's record. Checking the same jaw areas after compatible fillings have been placed you may find the jaw area that looked bad does not need surgery. Surgical sites need to be rechecked at each six month check up to be sure the jaws continue to be healthy.

Patient: "If you find a problem in the teeth or jawbone with CEDS, what do you do?"

Dentist: "A decision must be made by both the dentist and patient. Two things can be done for the tooth; 1) extraction or 2) a root canal. When a problem is in the teeth or jawbone, discovered through CEDS, the dentist and the patient together must make a decision as to whether a root canal or an extraction is the best course of action. Problems in the jawbone will need surgery to clear the infection.

Research has established that an unhealthy or dead tooth should be removed. Dead teeth can cause the loss of a body function. Refer to The Teeth and Body Energy chart to see the association of teeth to organ and tissue systems. Your dentist will be better equipped to help you if he has a working knowledge of conductance points, paired organs, and the meridian pathways. Today's computer software and on-screen graphics of the meridian pathways makes this an easy task for the dentist and physician to help patients with oral health concerns.

Case: Mary Ellen, age 58, muscle pain and fatigue.

Mary Ellen, an RN, noticed pain in the lower right jaw where she had no teeth. An x-ray did not show anything unusual in the bone. CEDS indicated an imbalance indicating possible pathology. Surgical exploration found a large cavitation where the CEDS showed an imbalance in the jaw.

Mary Ellen sent this thank you note. "Thank you for helping

me feel healthy again; my muscle aches and pains and fatigue are gone. I just feel so much better. I plan to do my neural therapy today to make sure the healing process goes well. Thank you, thank you, and thank you, Mary Ellen". Because of CEDS, Mary Ellen's problem was solved. Here again, energy dentistry made the difference.

Patient: "Do you send in a biopsy of infected teeth or jaw bone, and where do you send your biopsy for analysis?"

Dentist: "Biopsy tests will confirm any pathology and/or toxicity of the teeth or jaw bone." The best source for dental biopsies is:

The Surgical Pathology Service
Dr. Gerald Bouquot D.D.S.
University of Texas Dental Branch at Houston
Department of Diagnostic Sciences 30.94
6516 M.D. Anderson Blvd.
Houston, TX 77030
Phone: 713-500-4401
800-736-3098
- - to send biopsies or root canals for pathological evaluation

Patient: Ask your dentist to explain the procedures for replacing missing teeth.

Dentist: There are two methods of replacing missing teeth: 1) a bridge is fixed to the remaining teeth with bonding; 2) a removable partial can be made. Fixed bridges must be kept clean under the false tooth and around the supporting teeth, while removable partials can be removed for cleaning and flossing. Refer to Chapter 2 or chapter 10 for more information on bridges or partials/dentures.

Opting for a removable partial can also save money; should you lose an adjacent tooth, another tooth can easily be added to the partial. A second partial can come in handy if the first one breaks, or if your dog chews it up. My patient took his dentures out for an afternoon nap, placing them on the nightstand. He awakened to fine the dentures were gone. His dog had taken the dentures out in the back yard and buried them. And no, he could not find them. The next week I made my patient a new set of dentures, and the dog was forgiven. Well, not really!

Ask your dentist to explain his or her position on implants.

Mechanically, implants may be very good, however the biocompatibility of the implant material may not be. The question is: how does the patient feel after the implants have been in place for a period of time?

I have removed many implants because the signature, or energy, when measured with CEDS shows an imbalance. Patients indicate that they feel better after removal of the implant. Another consideration is the bacterial and protein toxins under the free margin of the gum, around the post of the implant. Gum tissue does not attach to the implant like it does to a natural tooth. Meticulous brushing and flossing is necessary if implants are placed. Frequent CEDS checks need to be done to determine the affect of the implant on the patient's organ systems. Very little is known about long term side effects from dental implant materials. The implanting of a metal implant base into the jawbone poses the risk of triggering an auto-immune reaction and the body may reject that material as foreign to it.

Reference: Dr. Boyd Haley U. of Kentucky www.iaomt.com

Refer to Chapter 8, Dr Eggleston's article on metals and how they affect our immune system.

Reference from Swedish Journal on Titanium call DAMS 1-800-311-6265

A variety of symptoms that mimic bacterial, viral and chemical health problems draw attention away from checking the teeth and jaws as the underlying cause. Remember what Dr. Voll said: 80 to 90 percent of systemic problems are caused, or influenced by the oral cavity. He often talked about the filling materials, root canals, abscessed teeth, and infections in the jaws as being major players in causing health problems. He also referred to hidden infections in the tonsils and sinuses. Patients today are looking for dental professionals who are aware that the oral cavity may be the cause of their poor health.

Dr. Cook's comment: I already told you about the patient that had over thirty years of facial pain. She had consulted thirty-three health professionals who had totally overlooked her mouth as a cause. Go to Chapter 13 for Mary Ann W.'s, story and recovery.

Chapter 20

Computerized Electro-Dermal Screening

CEDS uses computer graphics to display the readings. The dentist is able to customize a list of points as suggested in the software point detection section. Understanding that everything has energetic effects can alert us to our own health concerns as well as those of our patients.

Classes by the manufacturer cover the basic function of the CEDS. In the advanced class of "imbalanced readings", conductance points that do not balance with the manufacture's suggestions, look to the oral cavity to help find the answers. Initial examinations using CEDS normally show high readings with indicator drops due to metal fillings and infections in the oral cavity.

Computer software can be compared to an electrical circuit panel in your home. You can push breakers on a circuit panel to shut off electricity to different areas in your home. This principle is used with computer-stored remedies to block high readings and indicator drops related to the cause of patient's problems associated with the oral cavity.

Causes of imbalanced readings are the following: restorative metals, metal oxides and fluoride in composites, base metals with nickel, root canal infections, and dental gold, as well as pure gold in gold foil *fillings.*

The following will cause "imbalanced readings" when checking with CEDS:

Methylene blue in clothing labels, this blockage affects the nervous system and kidney function, ref: as mentioned in *Boericke's Materia Medica*. Petroleum in cosmetics as well as cadmium in women's cosmetics for rosy cheeks, hair spray or mousse, formaldehyde, DDT, chlordane, polio vaccine, microwaved water or food, barium, lead, base metals found in stainless crowns, partials, and surgical clips. Electrical radiation can be a big problem: electrical magnetic frequency, atomic radiation, fluorescent lights, electric heat and electric wiring in the walls. Car openers on a key chain in pockets and credit card magnetic strips in wallets are both problems. A hair piece or a wig that has synthetic fibers can cause high readings and indicator drops. Hair clips with a metal spring carry an electrical charge that can be detected with CEDS. Natural fiber clothing is important for obtaining balanced reading with CEDS; *have a cotton gown for your patient if clothing is an issue.*

Case: Ruth, age 40, CEDS unbalanced readings.

Ruth's conductance points could not be balanced during her electro-dermal screening exam. One vitamin pill in her pocket contained a toxic solvent (ethylene glycol). After removing the pill from her pocket, all high conductance points returned to normal.

Conductance points should be between 48 and 58 without an indicator drop. Balanced readings mean the patient can be checked for compatible filling material. I have found only three restorative materials sensitive patients can tolerate: Refer to Chapter 16 on Holistore, Premise Indirect (formally BelleGlass), and Vitalon 1060 for dentures, (Point 4 composite, Bistite II bonding material may be used in some cases).

Patients often feel a burst of energy after their mercury amalgams have been removed, but encounter fading of this good feeling after a short period of time. A possible reason for this energy loss is that compatible filling materials were not used to replace the mercury silver amalgam fillings.

Checking a tooth for vitality with CEDS requires removal of the filling down to the solid dentine. Remember, after removal of the mercury amalgams a bite wing x-ray can be taken to find any remaining filling. Leaving a speck of this amalgam in the tooth will produce the same bad energy as leaving the whole filling. Everyone has a different tolerance for metal and for composite fillings, as well as for infection in the oral cavity. Dead teeth, root canals and cavitations are usually the next layer of causes of health problems. CEDS helps find these major problems, making patients aware of the source of a current or pending health crisis.

Detoxification from heavy metal, pesticides, plastics, industrial pollution and nutrient-depleted foods has to be an ongoing effort for good health. Toxic materials can take a long time to surface and be recognized as the cause of health problems. Drinking half your body weight in ounces of clean water with one fourth teaspoon of sea salt is the simplest and least expensive detoxifying method. Visit www.watercure.com for more information on the importance of water.

Patient Preparation

It is extremely important to have a pH of 6.4 to 7.0 when removing mercury silver fillings. Premier Research Lab finds that with a pH in this range, minerals will coat the brush cells on the wall of the intestinal tract *with calcium*. Coral Legend minerals are designed to protect the intestinal wall from absorbing heavy metals. Contact www.prlabs.com or www.Healthlinecc.com. Premier Research Lab has a special clay and bath to help remove heavy metals from hands and feet; this clay opens up these "four doorways" for toxic metals to leave your body.

Urine and stool tests can be taken before and after using the clay to check the effectiveness of the removal of heavy metals from your body. I use Doctor's Data in Chicago (phone: 800-323-2784) for testing toxic metals. Check with a health care professional to order a test kit. Metametrix Laboratory is another lab for heavy metal testing, request a Cardio-ion panel, and Gastrointestinal Profile. A Porphyrin Profile will aid in finding specific heavy metals. Go to www.metametrix.com or phone 770-446-5483). Dr. Sherry Rogers' book, *The High Blood Pressure Hoax* discusses the use of Detoxamin to remove heavy metals.

An acidic condition caused by the Standard American Diet (SAD), which includes sugar, grains, and processed foods,) leaves people susceptible to infection. The lack of minerals in commercial produce adds to this acid condition, endangering the health of our body. By eating fresh, organic fruits and vegetables, our body will be returned to a balanced pH. (*The Body Ecology Diet*, by Donna Gates and *The pH Miracle for Weight Loss* by Robert O. Young, Ph.D.)

Use pH paper to check the first morning urine for an acid or alkaline pH reading. Good absorption of our minerals depends on the body's ph level. Being outside of the 6.4 to 7.0 range indicates a need for minerals. Premier Research Lab found when you are outside of the normal pH you can feel lousy, pessimistic, angry, irritable, fatigued, have no energy and have no desire to help others. Within the 6.4 to 7.0 range you are feeling great, optimistic, happy, joyful, full of energy, and have a desire to help others. Yet a urine pH test is seldom advised in a dental office. All patients should have a urine pH test two to six weeks before their appointment, and if necessary, bring their pH level into balance. A balanced pH will give their body the best chance to heal from metal removal, extractions, and cavitational surgery. To order the Daily pH Paper, call Daily Manufacturing Inc. at 1-800-868-0700 or go to their website www.daily-mfg.com.

Chapter 21

Body Health Dentistry

Call DAMS International 1043 Grand Ave, #137, St. Paul, MN 55105 phone: toll free from US and Canada 800-311-6265 for handouts, books on health and lists of knowledgeable dentists in your state or province.

Medical doctors will find their treatment is more effective when the oral cavity is free of the following: silver mercury amalgams, dental gold, nickel base metals, metal frameworks for partial dentures, dental implants, composites with metal oxides and fluoride, root canal filled teeth, dead teeth, cavitations (infection in the jaw bone), plastic denture base materials containing cadmium and the flexible plastics used in some partials.

Immune Systems and Metal Fillings.

Dr. Harold Kristal, D.D.S. did a thirty-patient study checking the blood immune panel of patients before and after the removal of metal fillings. Each case had an eighty to one hundred percent improvement of their immune system.

Dr. David Eggelston, D.D.S., published an article in The Prosthetic Journal showing the same result, that is, the immune system improved after the removal of nickel and amalgam restorations. He then replaced small amounts of mercury amalgam fillings inside the confines of these composite fillings, and found the immune system indicators showed a decrease by half. Read his article in Chapter 8.

Work that was done by Dr. Murray Vimy and Dr. Fritz Lorschieder at the University of Calgary medical school placed radioactive mercury in amalgam fillings in the teeth of test animals. Radioactive mercury ions that left the fillings were detected throughout the animals' bodies, with high concentrations mainly in the kidney and jaw tissue.

What is a Cavitation?

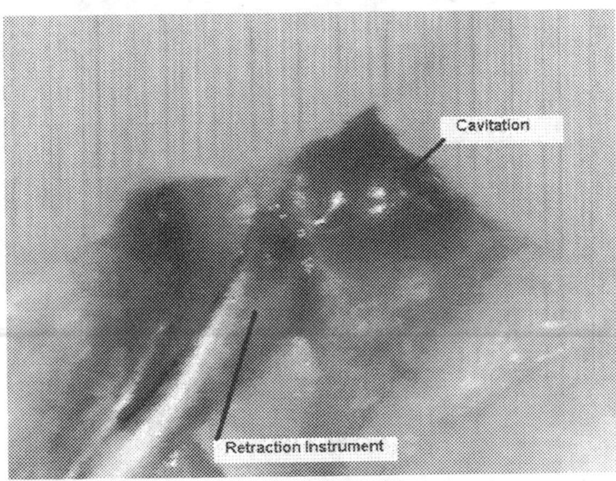

This is a cavitation

Cavitation is a term used to describe places inside the jawbone that are dead or dying. Biopsies of diseased jawbone have tested as being extremely toxic. Cavitations, in my experience, are often caused by the extraction of a tooth when incompatible filling materials are in other teeth. Remember the energy of the fillings and the patient's energy has to be compatible for good healing. All infections affect our health.

Because medical doctors know very little about the oral cavity, they may be prescribing medication for seemingly unrelated symptoms caused by fillings, infected teeth, or cavitations while overlooking the real cause. Dentists in general, need to know more about metal fillings and how the immune system can affect the health of their patient. Also, cavitations in the jaw are not always detected until weeks or months following an extraction. Cavitations can be cross checked with CEDS for symptoms in organ and tissue systems.

I have found CEDS to be more accurate than x-rays for detecting the exact location of infected teeth and jaws. Using the CEDS instrument makes jaw surgery more conservative, in that the dentist is able to find and remove only what is needed for a good result. Checking the same area with CEDS, eight to ten weeks after surgery, will determine if the surgery was successful.

Finding the source of facial pain is accomplished in different ways. Using local anesthetic to isolate the area of discomfort is one way to find where the pain is coming from. This may be painful for the patient due to the injections. Some dentists and oral surgeons use x-ray to locate the spots considered to be a cavitation in the jaws. Thermal imaging, Cavitat (ultrasonic scans), and CEDS are painless ways of finding trigeminal neuralgia and infection in jaws. Unlike CT scans, which deliver massive amounts of x-ray radiation into the bone and head, thermal imaging, the Cavitat and CEDS deliver no x-ray radiation at all and are therefore safer, as well as non-invasive. If surgery is necessary to remove infected bone, a biopsy is standard for confirming pathology.

How do we know when to check for cavitations?

CEDS, along with x-rays and oral exams, will become a standard procedure for finding cavitations. Many symptoms are caused by cavitations, dead teeth, and root canal treated teeth that go unnoticed for years. Finding the cause will help to eliminate pain and unnecessary medication. Infections and pain in the oral cavity are usually treated with antibiotics, anti-inflammatory medications), and pain killers. Such an approach may only mask symptoms, and may even cause new adverse side effects. Removal of wisdom teeth and cavitations can be very important to a patient's health.

Case: Rene Schneider, age 28, twelve years of pain.

Refer to tooth chart: Appendix B

Rene came to our office after twelve years of pain in her left jaw, sinus, and left ear. I checked her jaw on Ly2 with CEDS and found this conductance point a problem in areas # 1, # 3, # 24, and # 32. Later we found jaw pathology in areas # 16 and # 17. I performed cavitational surgery to remove the infection followed by re-testing with CEDS, and found no signs of infection. Rene confirmed the good results, she had no more pain.

Rene wrote this letter to Dr. Cook:

> "I wanted to say thank you to you all... I had such facial pain in my jaw, sinus and ear for 12 years. I was in a lot of pain. Trying to raise kids, be a wife and not to be crabby was very challenging! My pain started after I gave birth, many Doctors of all sorts said my pain was all in my head. They said you have TMJ, you have this or you have that.
>
> I became a Naturopath because of my pain and did lots of research. I did all of the cleanses, herbs, etc., and I was still getting terrible pain. So, I tried the last thing on my list, I came to Dr. Douglas Cook. I was scared because 1) He was another Doctor and what would he say, 2) How much more money do I have to dish out? As my husband pays the bills and I raise the kids. 3) Will this surgery work? 4) I have to convince my husband to drive me 400 miles with the kids and even though this surgery works, I wasn't convinced yet.

Dr. Cook was the only doctor that really listened to my pain and suffering, and could hear it. He proved and disproved what the other doctors said. Yes, it was all in my head and I don't have TMJ. Dr. Cook said let's do the easy stuff first then we will see what we have left over.

I cried tears of relief in his chair as he did the cavitational surgery, I could feel the burdens being lifted off in the dental chair, my palpitations went away, and years of weight was being pulled off. I am so grateful to Dr. Douglas Cook and the staff; they were so caring and helpful. I love them all. The money was nothing compared to having my life back. God bless him and his work."

Dr. Rene M. Schneider, Ph.D., N.D.

Removal of Wisdom Teeth

Removal of wisdom teeth is considered by the dental profession as a minor surgical procedure. But, removal of wisdom teeth is major surgery and should be treated accordingly. Preparation of the oral cavity before dental surgery requires replacement of all metal fillings and composites containing metal oxide, with compatible fillings to aid in complete healing. See section on dental materials in Chapter 16. After dental surgery with this protocol the patient will experience very little bleeding, very little swelling, and very little discomfort. After six months, a CEDS check of the surgical area should show a high percentage of healing with healthy bone and no sign of a cavitation (residual infection).

Chapter 22

Electro-Dermal Screening

Health Professionals Start Here

Dentists, as health care providers, know the oral cavity like no other health profession. With the use of CEDS, along with their knowledge and skills, they have a running start in helping many patients.

Published research proves that metals placed in our mouths are toxic. From this we can easily understand that metals and metal oxide fillings are a major part of this health burden. Patients exhibit a variety of health symptoms from these restorative materials as well as from root canals, dying teeth, infection in the jaws, and implants. Tonsils and sinuses also play an important role in symptoms commonly ascribed to food sensitivities. (Randolph, T. M.D., An Alternative Approach To Allergies, 1980.)

Metal fillings of different compositions have different effects, each having its own signature and energy influence. Silver amalgams containing mercury give off fumes when people chew or brush their teeth. Metal ions, though they affect patients both mentally and physically, are rarely mentioned as being a problem. Mercury vapor release from mercury silver amalgams can be seen on the eight minute DVD "Smoking

Teeth=Poisonous Gases". Contact DAMS at 800-311-6265 for a copy of this DVD.

Energy effects in dental materials are described in my patient case histories, in Chapter 12. Each case involves fillings and health problems resulting from the energy of incompatible dental materials

The article "Whole-body imaging of the distribution of mercury released from dental fillings into monkey tissues" (Hahn, L.J., Kloiber, R., Leininger, R.W., Lorschieder, F.L., and Vimy, M.J., 1990) explains how galvanic current releases the metallic ions from amalgam fillings that contain radioactive mercury. Amalgam tattoos are mercury solids that have been deposited into gum or cheek tissue. These tattoos provide visible evidence of mercury amalgams presence in the mouth.

A CEDS device quickly determines compatibility of dental materials and checks for infections as well. You can find the full article (Whole-body imaging - monkey tissues) and references by contacting the DAMS at 800-311-6265. Information can be found in the reference section of this book.

Dr. Voll, M.D., a genius who used electronics to find balances and imbalances, made an outstanding contribution with biofeedback through conductance or acupuncture points to determine health conditions. CEDS instruments send out a small signal to the patient's system through conductance points. In healthy patients, a reading of 50, on a scale of 0-100 will be sent back to the computer. This balanced reading of 50, plus or minus 4-6 points, should hold steady for 4-5 seconds, and indicates that the system is within a normal range of health.

If the reading goes higher than 50 and falls back 1 or more points, we will look for the patient to have health interferences. Readings above 50 usually indicate inflammation, the drop in the reading meaning that there is an additional burden to organ or tissue systems. I have listed in this chapter dental items that can change normal readings to abnormal readings.

Review these steps needed before you proceed to the next patient evaluation:

1. Know the contents of dental material.

2. Understand that everything has energy.

3. Understand the Teeth and Body Energy chart. Remember this chart is to remind us that each tooth is much more than just a hard surface in the oral cavity.

4. Limit yourself to those conductance points and organ systems related to the oral cavity, tonsils, and sinuses.

Every manufacturer of the CEDS biofeedback instrument conducts classes on its use, for example, the pressure needed on the conductance points for consistent readings and the location of these specific conductance points. Practice will give you a consistency of readings, and confidence in positioning the probe on the conductance points.

Health professionals can appreciate Dr. Voll's description of the indicator drop related to problems at a conductance point. He warned, "Watch for the one point drop; it can indicate health problems every bit as important as the big indicator drops."

High readings with an indicator drop can be caused from environmental toxins, pesticides, bacteria, viruses, incompatible fillings, as well as from jaw infections, and these causes must be considered with each patient. Be a detective! Ask your patient about other possibilities such as nutritional supplements, prescriptions, chemicals in their work place, food and water heated in a microwave; all are possibilities along with the above interferences.

A dentist must be aware of electro-magnetic frequencies and stray voltage, real problems to our health. Electrical currents that come from metal fillings in the teeth make CEDS cavitational readings look like pathology. Always check cavitation areas before and after the teeth have been restored, as cavitation surgery may not be necessary once dental materials have been changed.

Case: Betty, age 28, cavitations.

I held a two-day seminar for four dentists. One dentist brought a patient with him who had two cavitations according to CEDS, one on the lower right, and one on the lower left in the wisdom tooth areas.

I did the basic measuring on the conductance points Ly2 on the right and left hands. Each conductance point for the jaw had high readings with an indicator drop, suggesting incompatible dental filling material was the cause.

I looked over her full mouth x-ray with the four dentists. Both first and second lower molars on the left had composite fillings on the chewing surfaces containing fluoride, a toxic ingredient, and one molar had a small mercury amalgam under the composite. Her fillings were removed and replaced with Holistore, a non-metal oxide, non-fluoride composite, before cavitation surgery was done.

Following that, the patient's CEDS readings were perfect, indicating that what had appeared to be cavitations in the two wisdom teeth areas, was actually the effects of the filling materials. Removal of the fillings, and subsequent checking with CEDS revealed no pathology or infection, and no surgery was necessary.

Balanced readings with CEDS must be consistent on the lymph, nerve, circulation, and endocrine meridians, before selecting the most compatible dental materials. When testing questionable filling materials, a reading greater than fifty with an indicator drop suggests that the materials could cause a health problem.

It is important to look at everything as energy in order to understand how CEDS works with the body. Everything is made up of electrically charged particles. Combinations of these particles are either in balance or in conflict with our energy system. Any filling material a dentist uses must be compatible with the patient's energy system for the patient to maintain good health.

Cadmium is used to create the pink coloring in making the tissue-toned base for full dentures and partial dentures. Cadmium can cause a variety of symptoms easily overlooked by dentists and other health care professionals. Stainless steel partials can also cause problems due to the nickel in the alloy.

Case: John, age 73, joint pain.

John could only hunt and pick ginseng in his local woods by resting from time to time until the pain in his joints would settle. He would then move to another area, followed by another rest.

My father had placed masticators (stainless steel teeth) in John's lower denture sixteen years before he came to me. I checked the compatibility of the stainless steel with CEDS and found it to be a possible cause of the joint pain. Removal of the metal teeth completely relieved him of his joint pain in less than a week. He was so pleased that, two years later, he told me, "I've had more comfort in the past two years than in the last sixteen."

Case: George, age 61, extreme pain and fatigue.

George, a patient in our VA hospital, told his roommate, Fritz, about the pain and fatigue he felt at the end of each day. No medical doctor could figure out the cause. Fritz noticed George's upper stainless steel partial that he would take out at night, and asked George how he felt in the morning after having the partial out all night. George said he had no pain in the morning and didn't feel fatigued. Fritz asked George to leave the partial out for the rest of the day until the doctors made their rounds to check him. That evening, doctors asked George how he felt, and he told them "I feel better than I have in years." George told the doctors that "Dr. Fritz" had figured out that the cause of his pain and fatigue was the metal partial. George was off to the V.A. hospital dental clinic the next morning for an all plastic partial.

Case: Fritz, age 64, high blood pressure.

Fritz, the person mentioned in the previous case, had had high blood pressure before I removed his mercury silver amalgams. At each appointment I took Fritz's blood pressure. His blood pressure did not change until I replaced his stainless steel partial with an all-plastic partial. Compatible dental materials helped his blood pressure to normalize.

The cases about George and Fritz demonstrate how dental materials may be a primary cause of pain and of poor health. Knowing the content of dental materials can direct health practitioners to many patient problems. Along with x-rays and CEDS, Material Safety Data Sheets are a big help in evaluating affects of restorative dental materials.

Dental Gold

Dental gold, an alloy of gold and other metals, is a toxic material used to make crowns and other restorations. Pure gold or gold foil can also be a disturbance to the patient's health, the same as with the dental gold alloy. (See Chapter 8 for Case history about Dr. Dave's gold inlays and gold foil removal).

Dental gold has an affinity for mercury released from silver mercury amalgam fillings. High heat will greatly increase the release of mercury vapor from gold restorations that are contaminating it. Order the "Smoking Teeth=Poisonous Gases" DVD (DAMS Phone: 1 800-311-6265) and you can see this demonstrated in the video.

Dental materials in teeth, if visible on x-rays, contain a metal or a metal oxide. But fluoride, which is also undesirable, is a non-metal and doesn't reveal its presence through x-rays. CEDS, however, will find its presence.

Health problems of tooth-organ systems show up mainly because of dental infections and toxic dental materials (i.e., silver mercury amalgam fillings, dental gold, non-precious metal alloys containing nickel gallium or nickel beryllium, fluoride and metal oxides in composites). Checking the relationship of organs to teeth or teeth to organs is called "cross-checking" in CEDS. Cross-checking will find the source of trouble whether it comes from the tooth or the organ.

Conductance Points

1) Finding conductance points is the first step in learning about CEDS; the second step is obtaining consistent readings that are solid. A good health history is needed to find the teeth that are associated with organ problems; with this information, we are able to see the important relationship of teeth to patient health. In learning the Teeth and Body Energy chart, you will quickly begin to understand the paired organ systems associated with patient symptoms.

2) Specific data entered into the computer are called remedies, and can energetically cancel any metal fillings, an infected tooth, or infection in the jaw, producing a balanced reading on Ly2. Immediately check the corresponding organ conductance point, if there is a balanced reading, the organ is healthy with the tooth being the trouble-maker. We can now look to the tooth for an incompatible filling material, infection in the tooth, or an infected jawbone at that site.

3) Check Ly2 point on the right hand, which is related to the lymphatic drainage of the right upper and lower jaw, and the same, is true for the left hand and related jaws. A balanced

CEDS reading of Ly2 indicates healthy teeth and jaws; imbalance of Ly2 indicates a possible problem with the teeth or jaw.

Large intestine problems, for example, and a deep lung cough, share a common bond and are known as "paired organ systems". Notice other organ combinations shown on The Teeth and Body Energy chart. This chart will also show that a dead or dying tooth, can affect two organ systems at one time.

Two books helpful in understanding the importance of Computerized Electro-Dermal Screening are:

(1)*An Electro-dermal Analysis of Biological Conductance* by Vincent J. Speckhart, M.D. You can email him at bioconductance@verizon.net to order his book.

(2) www.redwingbooks.com for Dr. Voll's book, *Interrelations Of Odontons and Tonsils To Organs, Fields Of disturbance, and Tissue Systems*

These two books are important additions to your library for a basic understanding of meridians and conductance points for the oral cavity and the entire body.

Remember Dr. Voll's statement: "80 to 90 percent of systemic problems are caused or influenced by the oral cavity, tonsils, and sinuses." Dr. Voll's statement puts the dentist in an elite group of health care providers no other professional can claim!

For consistent results, follow these three steps to success with CEDS:

(1) Checking the tooth with CEDS after removal of a restoration will confirm that all incompatible filling material has been removed.

(2) Bite-wing x-rays will also confirm that all incompatible filling material has been removed.

(3) A final computerized electro-dermal screening will check the vitality of the tooth.

The Teeth and Body Energy chart is inserted in the back of this book.

Here is the Computerized Electro-Dermal Screening Protocol from my website www.dentistryhealth.com. The following information assumes the operator has a basic knowledge of computerized electro-dermal screening. Tooth location is numbered from upper right, to upper left, from lower left to lower right. They number from one to thirty-two.

Please refer to the Teeth and Body Energy chart, for the exact position of the teeth to those tissue systems that each tooth is related. A detailed knowledge of the chart is important in understanding the mouth and its relationship to your patient's health. The following procedure is used to evaluate the mouth and its energetic relationship to organs and tissue systems. Be aware of false negatives, the test says there is a problem when actually there is not a problem, and why a tooth may appear compromised due to outside interference fields. This protocol will also help to differentiate between dental materials and diseased teeth that cause abnormal signals.

Procedure:

Let us begin with an evaluation of a patient coming to the office for Computerized Electro-Dermal screening. Bring up the signal point screen or make your individual screen for dental checking. The conductance points I use will vary from two to three points for each meridian on one hand. These points are as follows: Ly 1, CMP Ly, Ly2, Lu 11, LU CMP, Lu 10.5, LI 1, CMP LI, LI 2, LI 3, LI 4, ND 1a, CMP ND, ND 3, Cir 9, CMP Cir, Al 1, CMP Al, Al 3, CMP OD, TW 1, CMP TW, TW 3, H 9, CMP H, H 8a, SI 1, CMP SI, SI 2. The purpose of these conductance points is to establish a base value for the meridians.

If you consistently see high readings with indicator drops (ID) of varying degrees this will indicate there is a problem in the oral cavity. One must balance these readings to between 48 and 55, and in most cases you will be able to balance to 50 without an indicator drop. To balance these points, you must become a good detective and find the reason or reasons for the imbalances in the readings.

The following materials are ranked from greatest to least in terms of how they affect body energy: mercury silver fillings (amalgams), non-precious crowns and bridges (made from nickel, chrome, and beryllium, or nickel chrome, gallium, and molybdenum). Remedies are in the dental nosodes, energy of the actual material. Aluminum oxide is in most composites, along with iron oxide and fluoride. Some composites contain barium; however barium is more likely to be found in dental cavity liners, such as Hypocal (slak lime) or calcium hydroxide. Gold Zahngold or dental gold is made of many alloys and is never pure gold. Cadmium is a heavy metal found in gutta-percha, (used in filling root canal treated teeth) and in the pink plastic base of dentures and partial dentures. Partials and implants have an effect on the CEDS readings due to the electric charge in the metal.

Be aware of amalgam tattoos that may result from galvanic current transferring metallic ions into the tissue. These tattoos can also help produce the patient's imbalanced conductance point readings.

Note: See Chapter 4 for the case study on Sally, who had an amalgam tattoo on her palate.

It is important to know the effect of interferences that can cause an imbalance to ND 1a, Ly 1, Cir 9 and Tw 1 points. Cosmetics, medications, and a variety of items used or worn by a patient, are some examples of interferences. Each interference can be blocked, or canceled by entering a specific remedy into the computer, enabling the practitioner to balance these conductance points.)

The following is a list of items and materials that can cause an imbalance in the conductance points, in the computer is the remedy, for each interference.

1. cosmetics are usually petroleum-based; the remedy is petroleum 3x or 6x
2. hair permanents can contain formaldehyde; the remedy is formaldehyde 3x or 6x
3. labels in clothing; the remedy is methylene blue 3x or 6x
4. synthetic clothing; the remedy is polyacrylate 3x or 6x
5. fingernail polish; the remedy is iron oxide and/or petroleum
6. breast implants; use a remedy from the same material (silicone)
7. artificial joints made from nickel or use a remedy from the same material
8. wig caps sometimes contain nylon; the remedy is acrylate 3x or 6x, or remove the wig
9. TMJ implants; the remedy is autoacrylate 3x or 6x
10. medication that is not compatible, a remedy must be obtained
11. surgical clips or staples; the remedy is nickel or niccolum, which is German for nickel
12. supplements check ethylene glycol, a toxic substance used in preparing supplements
13. reinforcing pins in teeth (Whale Dent, a trade name); the remedy is nickel
14. root canal fillings; the remedy is cadmium or calcium hydroxide
15. bimetal currents from restorations in the teeth. Check with the Oral Potential Meter II instrument, http://www.metalpoison.net
16. electric blankets and heaters in water beds, the remedy is: aqua Hz 60 cycle AC
17. water beds; the remedy is polyvinylchloride or autoacrylate

The following is a list of items that can cause an imbalance in the conductance points, and should be removed prior to checking the patient with CEDS.

1. jewelry, either nickel-based or gold plated
2. ear rings, including those with plastic posts
3. hair pins
4. metal in the frames bows of eyeglasses. Graphite or all plastic frames seem to work better. Have patient bring in several types of frames and measure them with CEDS to find the most compatible pair for them.
5. electric watches, watches with stainless steel backs, and metal watch bands
6. shoes
7. contact lens and cleaner; remove lenses
8. chromic suture material
9. credit cards; the magnetic strips are an interference
10. car openers, pagers, cell phones

You will find other influences from environmental conditions in your area that have to be blocked in order to obtain balanced readings. When balancing of ND1a you can check other meridians and points that gave a high reading and indicator drop (ID's). If you have a balance on other points you know the oral cavity and the above list are the cause of high readings and ID's. Points that may not balance are control measurement points (CMP) for the heart and small intestine normally related to Ly2, (the jaw and wisdom teeth). You will have to check out the odontons, and balance Ly2 with jaw nosodes, then cross check the heart and small intestine to locate the problem. Balance of the heart and small intestine will tell you the odontons are the cause of the imbalance.

The next two steps will be helpful in locating the odonton that is causing an imbalance and the type of dental materials that appear to be most compatible. ND 1a is used to check dental restorative materials after it has been balanced with the above mentioned information. Patients can hold the restorative material or place it on the CEDS plate for checking compatibility.

Only two dental materials are consistently compatible, Premise Indirect (formally BelleGlass) neutral (no shade) and Holistore. Holistore is used for bonding and for small fillings. Both Holistore and Premise Indirect are a pleasing light shade; I have found most patients are more interested in their health than in appearances. I am always looking for other compatible restorative and bonding materials. Check my web site for the latest materials that may help your patients http://www.dentistryhealth.com.

Follow this step by step method for finding infection in the teeth and jaws. Ly2 (conductance point for the upper and lower jaw) when out of balance one of the following remedies, or nosodes, are used to balance this point, chronic Kiefer ostitis, gangrenous pulp, exudative ostitis, zahnsackchen, chronic bacterial ostitis, or chronic pulpitis. Generally four or more of the same remedy are needed to balance Ly2. Once Ly2 is balanced, stimulate on the gum (with an instrument) by pressing lightly on the jaw area or tooth above or below where you want to test. CEDS will give a high reading on Ly2 indicating a problem in the jaw or tooth. Test the teeth without any fillings to check their vitality with CEDS. Adding the compatible restorative material by placing it in the HOLD tank or on the plate will balance Ly2. This method is also used to evaluate the possibility of different filling materials under a crown. A balance, when the restorative material remedy is placed in the HOLD tank, indicates the tooth is healthy; an amalgam under a crown or inlay will cause an imbalance. Perform a final check of the tooth after it has been cleared of restorative or temporary fillings.

The location of cavitations is done in a similar manner by balancing Ly2 with one of the above mentioned nosodes. Following the procedure outlined above, stimulate the edentulous area and then measure Ly2. A balanced reading indicates healthy bone, a high reading and an indicator drop will mean a possible focal infection or cavitation. When checking several teeth or bony areas such as the wisdom teeth or where the wisdom teeth were, keep adding the nosode for Ly2 until you have gone through the mouth. As many as 50 or more odonton remedies may be placed in the hold tank to obtain a balance of Ly2. If there is pathology in the jawbone, surgery should be done and a biopsy sent to an oral pathologist or to Dr. Gerald Bouquot D.D.S. His address is on page 105 and 133.

If a dentist does not feel qualified or prepared to treat the cavitation himself, he should refer the patient to a practitioner who can locate and surgically treat it.

CEDS testing is invaluable in checking the surgical site before and after surgery, as it allows the surgeon to be conservative, and remove only the portion of the bone that is necessary to clear infection.

Finding an unhealthy tooth means you have to decide to either do a root canal or remove the tooth. However, the final decision should be made by the informed patient. Provide the patient with the following references:

The Root Canal Cover Up Exposed! by Dr. George Meinig, D.D.S.

Dr. Boyd Haley's has transferred peer review articles on root treated teeth to the web site www.iaomt.com.
The Price Pottenger nutritional foundation, www.price-pottenger.org has valid root canal research articles by Dr. Weston Price.

Case: Grace, age 54, suicidal.

Grace tried to commit suicide by walking out on a frozen river behind her house. After she fell into the cold water, she changed her mind. Her neighbor saw her and ran to the river with his boat, to save her. Good job, neighbor.

Grace's x-rays showed root canals with many metal restorations, which pointed to a possible cause of her depression. I suggested removing her metals fillings and replacing them with compatible composites, leaving no metal or metal oxide composites in her mouth. Next, I removed the root canals.

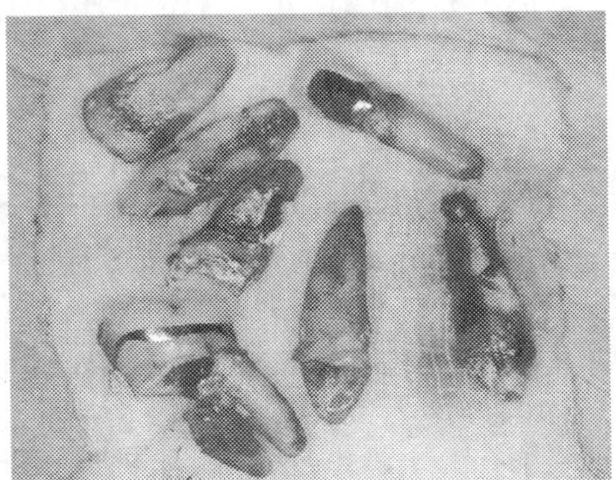

Photograph of her root canal treated teeth

At her financial convenience, I will change the Holistore fillings in high stress chewing areas to a more durable restoration. Two all-plastic, heat-cured partials replaced her missing teeth for good looks and chewing. Grace is now working two jobs and has regained the energy she had lost.

Chapter 23

Dry Socket - Cause and Treatment

Definition: a **dry socket** is an open extraction site that does not heal. It results in pain that is not stopped by strong medication. The health of the patient and the presence of metal fillings in other teeth seem to be factors that may cause a dry socket. There is a consistent odor and taste to all dry sockets along with the severe pain that becomes evident within forty-eight hours after an extraction. Dry sockets can cause jawbone cavitations and other health problems.

Infection is the most immediate and apparent cause of a dry socket and the dentist's removal of all toxic and infected tissue at the extraction site is important. Homeopathics and other anti-infective measures help prevent or fight off infection. A severe new pain in hours or days after an extraction usually means infection.

In most cases, good healing after the removal of a tooth is dependent on having compatible fillings in the remaining teeth. It is the same with any oral surgery, when compatible filling materials have been used there will be very little bleeding, very little swelling and very little discomfort after the procedure.

Relief from Dry Sockets - What to Do

The standard method of treating a dry socket is to re-open the site and surgically clean the socket, then pack the socket with iodoform gauze to start the healing process. Next, administer antibiotics and strong pain medication for the comfort of the patient.

But the simplest and most effective treatment for a dry socket is to use equal parts of a liquid containing Guaiacol, Peruvian Balsam, and Glycerin. Gently shake this mixture until completely mixed. Using a small piece of cotton the size of a grain of wheat, soak half of the cotton and remove the excess by blotting. Carefully place the cotton directly to the bottom of the dry socket, and set a timer for ten minutes. The pain will be relieved, and the patient will experience a warm, comfortable feeling.

The first treatment with dry socket medication is good for six to eight hours. Follow this period by treating again to continue the pain relief. Use this medication once every 24 hours for the next three to four days, or as needed. Remember, this socket should be tested with CEDS for a possible cavitation in six to eight weeks.

If the pain does not stop, there are two possible reasons: 1) either the piece of cotton is too large, having expanded when wet, and causing pain, or 2) the socket has two or more roots and both need to be treated to the full depth of the site. No anesthetic is necessary, thus the patient can tell in ten minutes if the pain has gone away. The patient can also tell when they feel the treated cotton deep enough in the socket. Patient feedback is important for proper placement of the cotton.

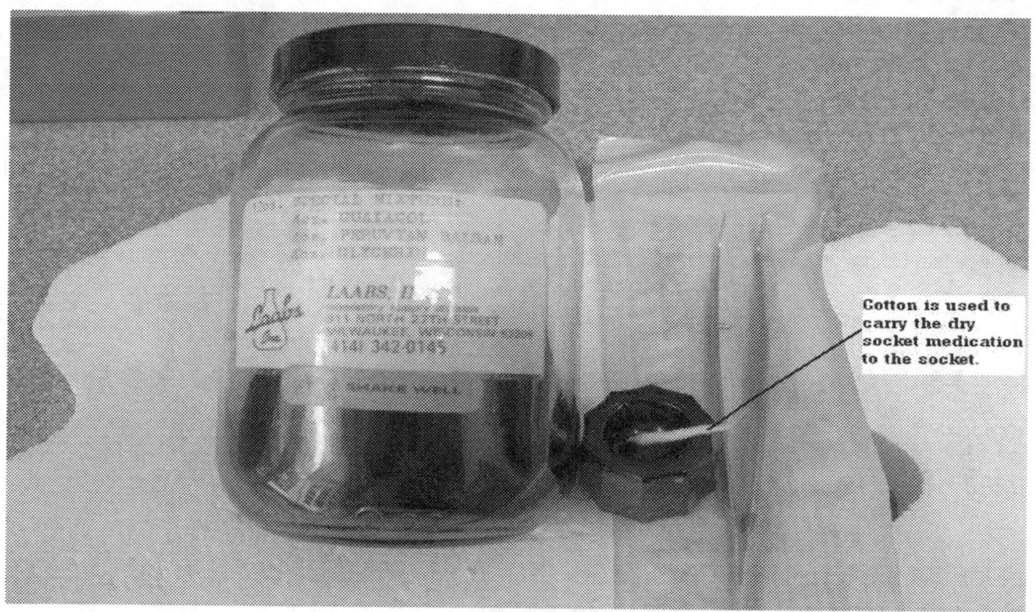
Cotton is used to carry the dry socket medication to the socket.

Dry socket medication, tweezers, small well and cotton.

For patients who live some distance from the office, I will make up a kit with everything they may need to treat themselves. All previously healed dry socket sites that I have checked with CEDS and surgically biopsied have proved to be infected.

My father learned this procedure from an oral surgeon in 1920. He had consistently good results with this procedure, and I have had the same good results for every dry socket I have treated. Thanks, Dad.

Chapter 24

Build, Not Destroy, Your Practice

Patient comfort is basic in building a practice. Every dentist needs to put him or herself in the dental chair to have a tooth worked on once a week as a reminder of the care patients would like to have from them. Use of a buckwheat-seed horseshoe pillow covered with a cotton towel will support the patient's neck while in the dental chair. This small comfort has elicited favorable comments from patients.

Anesthesia is one of the keys to success with all patients, and anesthetics have a profound effect when not compatible. Anytime chemicals are administered to a patient there will be effects, however using an anesthetic without a preservative and without a vasoconstrictor adds to its compatible qualities.

A vasoconstrictor has a downside. It is designed to constrict blood vessels to hold anesthetic and keep the tooth pain free for a longer time. But in slowing the blood supply to the area of an extracted tooth, vasoconstrictors delay healing by not allowing the blood to enter the surgical site immediately. Preservatives in anesthetics are toxic to our organs. My choice of an anesthetic is 3% Polocaine by Dentsply. You can order at www.dentsply.com or through your dental supplier. Polocaine is a short acting anesthetic for operative and surgical procedures on the upper and lower jaws. Needles used to inject the anesthetic are another key to comfort for the patient. I use 30-

gauge, short needles for all injections. Patients will let you know when they need additional anesthetic.

Talking to a recent graduate from dental school, I realized he needed help using anesthetics on his patients. Injecting into the infra-orbital foramen is not a procedure patients enjoy. Injection in the palate for removing a tooth needs to be done close to the tooth being removed. Patients will be more comfortable with only the injections needed to get the job done.

Injections to remove upper teeth need to be done in the soft tissue slightly anterior to the tooth being prepared for a restoration or removal, without touching the periosteum (a layer of tissue that covers the jaw bone). An injection in which the needle is forced under the periosteum is painful after the anesthetic comes out.

If the anesthetic does not relieve the pain in the time it takes to prepare for the surgery, use an anesthetic injection into the periodontal ligament. Or do the X tip Drill and Guide sleeve for interosseous introduction of the anesthetic directly through the jaw bone for the tooth's nerve. Heavy thick jaw bone makes the interosseous technique difficult and it should be avoided if this is the case.

For teeth that do not become completely numb, an anesthetic can be introduced directly into the root canal, for optimal pain control.

Use the mental foramen to anesthetize the lower anterior teeth including the bicuspids. Anesthesia in this area works quickly for operative or surgical procedures. Extractions in this lower anterior area will require injections on the lingual jaw tissue of the tooth being removed.

Detoxification of the anesthetic can be accomplished with three to four thousand milligrams of vitamin C, after an appointment. Inform your patients not to take vitamin C for forty eight hours prior to the appointment. Vitamin C before an appointment may make the anesthetic less effective.

Appendix A

Environmental Dentistry (Instrumentation)

Testing equipment:

Computerized Electro-dermal Screening instruments:

Synergy Energy Systems
1223 Wilshire Blvd #321
Santa Monica CA 90403
Contact person, Jim Jose phone: 310-394-6497

Startech Health
1219 South 1840 West
Orem, UT 84058
Contact person, Bill Clark phone: 801-229-2500

Meter for Measuring Oral Galvanism II ion release, and for detecting caries:

Pertec Of Wisconsin Inc.
10971 Clinic Road
Suring WI 54174
Contact person, Dr. Doug or Dr. Bruce Cook, Phone: 920-842-2083, www.metalpoison.net

KaVo Intramatic LH
Cellular Optic Low Speed System, Air only and Electric hand piece produces EMF that can cause health problems.
Call 1-888-KaVo USA for a catalog

Standard Low Speed Operative Systems by KaVo
Head 80LD 1:1 Transmission Friction grip head
Contra Angle Attachment 20LH 1:1 transmission separate internal air/water
Speed range with air up to 20,000 rpm.

Motor Universal "E" Type 181L INTRA Air LUX Motor with Light speed range from 5,000 up to 20,000 rpm
Straight Low Speed Hand piece
Air driven speed up to 20,000rpm
Hand piece 10LH 1:1 Transmission with separate internal air/water coolant. Perfect for surgical reduction of buccal bone over the roots, separating the roots from the crown to roll the roots and tooth out.

The Surgical Pathology Service
Dr. Gerald Bouquot D.D.S.
University of Texas Dental Branch at Houston
Department of Diagnostic Sciences 30.94
6516 M.D. Anderson Blvd.
Houston, TX 77030
Phone: 713-500-4401
800-736-3098
- to send biopsies or root canals for pathological evaluation

Educational Resources for the Public - Dental Patients

DAMS (Dental Amalgam Mercury Solutions)
1043 Grand Ave, #317
St Paul, MN 55105

Call DAMS at 800-311-6265, which is toll-free from anywhere in the US or Canada.
DAMS will send out, upon request, a Dental-Health Guide on the dental amalgam mercury issue and other ways dentistry may affect health. With this guide, you will also receive a list of knowledgeable dentists and doctors in your state or province. The guide covers issues ranging from the protocol for safe amalgam removal, discussion of dental material choices, detoxification from mercury and other heavy metals, fluoride and

more. In addition to selling dozens of books and videos and having a periodic publication for DAMS members (ask for a sample issue), DAMS offers a public help line for people wanting to talk to a real person. To order any of these things or just to discuss your questions, call DAMS at 800-311-6265.

Educational Resources mainly for Biological Dentists or other Health Professionals or Scientists

These academies have memberships and hold conferences that are open to dentists, other health professionals, and scientists. Unfortunately, these conferences are not open to the general public.

IAOMT - International Academy of Oral Medicine and Toxicology
8298 Champions Gate Blvd, #193
Champions Gate, FL 33896
863-420-6373 www.iaomt.org

Holistic Dental Association
619-923-3120 www.holisticdental.org

Sources for Dental Products And Materials

DEMI - a high powered ultra-violet light that is used to set the dental material
Kerr Corporation
3235 Deming Way
Middleton WI 53562

Dental Lite - a light that the doctor wears on his glasses to see in the mouth

Designs for Vision Inc.
760 Koehler Ave
Ronkonkoma, NY 11779

Thermal Life Far Infrared Sauna
High Tech Health
800-794-5355 www.hightechhealth.com

Hydro Floss - An Oral Irrigator that helps remove debris that remain after brushing/flossing
404 Business Center Drive
Birmingham, AL 35244
1-800-635-3594
www.hydrofloss.com

Oratec - Sub gingival Hand Held Irrigator helps remove debris from in between the teeth
Perio Flex
12181 Balls Ford Road
Manassas, VA 20109
1-800-368-3529
www.oratec.net

Dental Health Products Inc.
2614 North Sugar Bush Road
P.O. Box 176
New Franken, WI 54229
1-800-626-2163

- 3M ScotchBond Multi-Purpose # 2 Primer
- 3M ScotchBond Multi-Purpose # 3 Adhesive
- 3M ESPE Durelon Cement (Temporary Cement)
- 3M ESPE Durelon Liquid
- Polocaine - anesthetic (or you can order it through Dentsply (www.dentsply.com)
- Cavitron - Ultra-sonic Scaling Unit
- Bistite II DC - Manufacture: Tokuyama Corp. Dist: J. Morita USA, Inc. Check with CEDS for compatibility

Den-Mat
2727 Sky Way Drive
Santa Maria, CA 93455
1-800-433-6628

- Tenure A Adhesive
- Tenure B Adhesive
- Tenure S Bond Enhancer
- Dry Bond
- Holistore A Slow Set (in a red container)
- Holistore B Slow Set (in a blue container)
    - mix the Holistore A and B together to get your filling or bonding material

Kerr Corporation
1717 West Collins Ave
Orange, CA 92867
1-800-537-7123

- Point 4 check patient with CEDS for compatibility
- Opti-Bond Solo Plus
- Gel Etchant (purple in color)
- Premise Indirect (formally Belleglass) (neutral and shaded) Many labs will not make neutral. Contact Cook Lab. 920842-2083 for neutral or shaded restorations.

Ellman International Inc.
1135 Railroad Ave
Hewlett, NY 11557
1-800-835-5355

- Hypo-Cal without barium (available on order)

Cooley & Cooley Ltd.
Houston, TX 77041
www.copalite.com

- Copalite

Appendix B

Teeth And Body Energy Chart

The energetic relations of teeth (or odontons) with respect to organs and tissue systems

Endocrine glands		Anterior pituitary lobe	Para-thyroid	Thyroid	Thymus	Posterior pituitary lobe	Inter-mediate pituitary lobe	Pineal gland		Pineal gland		Posterior pituitary lobe	Inter-mediate pituitary lobe	Thymus	Thyroid	Para-thyroid	Anterior pituitary lobe
Sense organs		Internal ear Tongue	Tongue		Nose		Eye, posterior portion	Nose		Nose		Eye, posterior portion	Nose		Tongue		Internal ear Tongue
Paranasal sinuses			Maxillary sinus		Ethmoid cells		Sphenoidal sinus	Frontal sinus		Sphenoidal sinus / Frontal sinus			Ethmoid cells		Maxillary sinus		
Joints		Shoulder ul. s. Elbow ul. s. Hand, ulnar side / Foot, plantar side Toes / Sacro-iliac joint	Jaw / Anterior hip Anterior knee Medial ankle joint		Shoulder ra. s. Elbow ra. s. Hand, radial side / Foot Big toe		Posterior knee / Hip / Ankle joint / lateral	Sacro-coccygeal joint / posterior		Posterior knee / Sacro-coccygeal joint / Ankle joint / posterior		Hip / lateral	Shoulder ra. s. Elbow ra. s. Hand, radial side / Foot Big toe		Jaw / Anterior hip Anterior knee Medial ankle joint		Shoulder ul s Elbow ul s. Hand, ulnar side / Foot, planter side Toes / Sacro-iliac joint
Segments of the spinal marrow and Dermatomes		SC2 SC1 STh1 SC8 STh7 STh6 STh5 SS2 SS1	SC2 SC1 STh12 STh11 SL1		SC2 SC1 SC5 SC6 SC7 STh2 STh3 STh4 SL4 SL5		SC2 SC1 STh8 STh9 STh10	SC2 SC1 SL3 SL2 SCo SS5 SS4 SS3		SC1 SC2 SL2 SL3 SS3 SS4 SS5 SCo		SC1 SC2 STh8 STh9 STh10	SC1 SC2 SC5 SC6 SC7 STh2 STh3 STh4 SL4 SL5		SC1 SC2 STh11 STh12 SL1		SC1 SC2 SC8 STh1 STh5 STh6 STh7 SS1 SS2
Vertebrae		C2 C1 TH1 C7 Th7 Th6 Th5 S2 S1	C2 C1 Th12 Th11 L1		C2 C1 C7 C6 C5 Th4 Th3 Th2 L5 L4		C2 C1 Th8 Th9 Th10	C2 C1 L3 L2 Co S5 S4 S3		C1 C2 L2 L3 S3 S4 S5 Co		C1 C2 Th8 Th9 TH10	C1 C2 C5 C6 C7 Th3 Th4 L4 L5		C1 C2 TH11 TH12 L1		C1 C2 C7 TH1 Th5 Th6 Th7 S1 S2
Organs		Heart, right side	Pancreas		Lung, right side		Liver, right side	Kidney, right side		Kidney, left side		Liver, left side	Lung, left side		Spleen		Heart, left side
		Duodenum, right side Terminal ileum	Oesophagus Stomach, right side		Large intestine, right side		Gall-bladder Biliary ducts right side	Urinary bladder, right side Genito-urinary area Rectum, Anal canal		Urinary bladder, left side Genito-urinary area Rectum, Anal canal		Biliary ducts, left side	Large intestine, left side		Oesophagus Stomach, left side		Duodenum, left side Jejunum Ileum
Tissue systems		Central nervous system Limbic system															Central nervous system Limbic system
Other systems			Mammary gland, right side											Mammary gland, left side			
Jaw sections	upper	V.	IV.		III.		II.	I.		I.		II.	III.		IV.		V.	upper
American nomenclature		1	2	3	4	5	6	7	8	9	10	11	12	13	14	15	16	
International nomenclature		18	17	16	15	14	13	12	11	21	22	23	24	25	26	27	28	
Teeth diagram	right																	left
Tooth number		8+	7+	6+	5+	4+	3+	2+	1+	+1	+2	+3	+4	+5	+6	+7	+8	

Tooth number		8–	7–	6–	5–	4–	3–	2–	1–	–1	–2	–3	–4	–5	–6	–7	–8	
Teeth diagram	right (retro-molar)																	(retro-molar) left
International nomenclature		48	47	46	45	44	43	42	41	31	32	33	34	35	36	37	38	
American nomenclature		32	31	30	29	28	27	26	25	24	23	22	21	20	19	18	17	
Jaw sections	lower	V.	IV.		III.		II.	I.		I.		II.	III.		IV		V.	lower
Other systems		Energy exchange			Mammary gland right side								Mammary gland, left side				Energy exchange	
Tissue systems		Peripheral nerves	Arteries	Veins	Lymph vessels									Lymph vessels	Veins	Arteries	Peripheral nerves	
Organs		Terminal ileum Ileo-cecal area	Large intestine, right side		Oesophagus Stomach right side Pylorus Pyloric antrum		Gall-bladder Biliary ducts, right side	Rectum Anal canal Urinary bladder, right side genito-urinary area		Rectum Anal canal Urinary bladder, left side genito-urinary area		Biliary ducts, left side	Oesophagus Stomach left side		Large intestine, left side		Jejunum Ileum, left side	
		Heart, right side	Lung, right side		Pancreas		Liver, right side	Kidney, right side		Kidney left side		Liver, left side	Spleen		Lung, left side		Heart, left side	
Vertebral		C 2 C1 Th1 C7 Th7 Th6 Th5 S2 S1	C 2 C1 C7 C6 C5 Th4 Th3 L5 L4		C 2 C1 Th12 Th11 L1		C 2 C1 Th8 Th9 Th10	C 2 C1 L3 L2 S5 S4 S3 Co		C1 C2 L2 L3 S3 S4 S5 Co		C1 C2 Th8 Th9 Th10	C1 C2 Th11 Th12 L1		C1 C2 C5 C6 C7 Th3 Th4 L4 L5		C1 C2 C7 Th1 Th5 Th6 Th7 S1 S2	
Segments of the spinal marrow and Dermatomes		SC2 SC1 STh1 SC8 STh7 STh6 STh5 SS2 SS1	SC2 SC1 Sc7 SC6 SC5 STh4 STh3 STh2 SL5 SL4		SC2 SC1 STh12 STh11 SL1		SC2 SC1 STh8 STh9 STh10	SC2 SC1 SL3 SL2 SCo SS5 SS4		SC1 SC2 SL2 SL3 SS4 SS5 SCo		SC1 SC2 STh8 STh9 STh10	SC1 SC2 STh11 STh12 SL1		SC1 SC2 SC5 SC6 SC7 STh2 STh3 STh4 SL4 SL5		SC1 SC2 SC8 STh1 STh5 STh6 STh7 SS1 SS2	
Joints		Shoulder – Elbow, right side			Anterior hip Anterior knee		Posterior knee			Posterior knee			Anterior hip Anterior knee		Shoulder – Elbow, left side			
		Hand, ulnar side Foot, plantar side Toes	Hand, radial side Foot Big toe		Medial ankle joint		Hip	Sacro-coccygeal joint		Sacro-coccygeal joint		Hip	Medial ankle joint		Hand, radial side Foot Big toe		Hand, ulnar side Foot, plantar side Toes	
		Sacro-iliac joint			Jaw		Ankle joint lateral	Ankle joint posterior		Ankle joint posterior		lateral	Jaw				Sacro-iliac joint	
Paranasal sinuses			Ethmoid cells		Maxillary sinus			Frontal sinus		Frontal sinus			Maxillary sinus		Ethmoid cells			
							Sphenoidal sinus			Sphenoidal sinus								
Sense organs		Middle external ear Tongue	Nose		Tongue		Eye, anterior portion	Nose		Nose		Eye, anterior portion	Tongue		Nose		Middle external ear Tongue	
Endocrine glands						Gonad		Adrenal gland		Adrenal gland		Gonad						

Appendix C

Definitions

Abscess - a localized collection of pus in any part of the body, formed by tissue disintegration by an inflamed area. A tooth abscess is rotting bone tissue next to the root of a tooth, often caused by infection that has killed a tooth or by the infection and toxins released from a root canal treated tooth. Most often, a tooth abscess is suspected because of pain and is confirmed by an x-ray taken of the tooth (or teeth). However, an abscess might not be visible from the view of the tooth taken by a single x-ray; it might, in fact, be hidden between roots or behind a root. CEDS helps overcome this limitation by testing the tooth energetically. The TOPAS (now called HALITOX) test will also likely show serious bacterial and fungal infection at such a tooth. If an abscessed tooth is just root canal treated, what is going to take care of the abscess? The abscessed tooth should be extracted, with the diseased, abscessed area thoroughly cleaned out. CEDS can help determine that the surgical clean-out has been complete and successful.

Amalgam - any of the various mixtures of mercury with other metals. A dental amalgam is, by definition, a mixture of mercury with other metals which is soft enough to place and shape, but will then) harden into a durable filling. In dental amalgams, mercury is always about 50% of the new amalgam filling materials. The other metals are silver, copper, tin and a trace amount (less than 1%) of zinc. Amalgam manufacturer warning labels have a poison warning, a skull and crossbones symbol) about this product, indicating) that the product contains mercury, which causes neurological and kidney problems, and vision impairment. Sadly, most dental patients never see the product warning labels, and dentists often fail to tell them about the warning – it would scare them. The mercury content in old amalgam fillings has been measured at as low as 28% mercury, down from the original 50% mercury. (Eichman, R) That difference is explained by the vaporization of mercury from the amalgam's surface and through other pathways. The amalgam serves as a time-released poison for any patient with this type of filling material.

Amalgam tattoo - a solid mercury compound, usually black or blue in color, that has been deposited on the gum or check tissue inside the mouth. The compound may be, for example, mercury sulfide, which forms when hydrogen sulfide from bad breath reacts with mercury vapor or mercury ions given off by the amalgam fillings in the mouth. Amalgam tattoo removal should be carefully done by the dentist as part of the dental revision work done for the health-conscious patient.

Bridge - Sometimes bridges are supported by crowned teeth that are the abutment teeth (holding up the bridge). But crowning the abutment teeth just to have them hold up a bridge tends to unnecessarily weaken them: crowning involves a loss of enamel on all sides of the tooth. So, if a bridge is going to be placed, it is better to just bond the bridge onto the supporting abutment teeth.

CEDS - (**C**omputerized **E**lectro-**D**ermal **S**creening) A bio-feedback instrument that aids the dentist in finding the most compatible dental materials, and in locating infection in teeth and jaws.

Chelation - the ingestion of a substance, usually a drug, to chemically bind mercury or other heavy metals having more than one chemical bond, in order to detoxify the system. Currently, there are only three drugs that are used for heavy metal chelation detox for dental patients: DMPS, DMSA, and EDTA. The use of these drugs is controversial and they have been criticized for causing adverse side effects, especially when used at higher doses and on sicker, more fragile people. Today, there are an increasing number of detoxification methods which do not rely on the use of drugs and which are (technically speaking) not chelators. These detox methods may involve supplements and "skin methods" such as the use of bathing clays, Epsom salt baths and saunas followed by showering. (See "detoxification")

Detoxification - the process of removing toxins, such as mercury, lead, arsenic, fluoride, etc, from the body's internal organs,) and the brain. There are many approaches to detoxification (called "detox," for short) and they may involve supplements, "skin methods," such as Epsom salt baths, bathing clays, saunas, etc, as well as drugs, which are being used less frequently today, due to the availability of gentler, more natural methods. Diet and lifestyle also matter and certain foods have been found to be very helpful while other foods are best avoided. Contact DAMS for its Information Guide for information on current detox ideas and books on this important subject.

Endodontist - a dentist who specializes in the performance of root canal treatment of teeth that are dying or dead. Endodontics is the field of dentistry that specializes in the performance of "root canals," i.e. the root canal treatment of teeth. However, root canal treatments are also performed by general dentists, and not just endodontists. Read Root Canal Cover Up Exposed by George Meinig, D.D.S.

Fluoride - a combination of fluoride, a non-metal element, with another element such as sodium, aluminum or hydrogen. In general, the fluoride salts are highly poisonous. Sodium fluoride, for example, used in most drug store toothpastes, has been used as a rat poison and an insecticide. As used in tooth pastes or mouth rinses, sodium fluoride is very effective at killing bacteria. However, some of the fluoride used in such dental applications is swallowed or otherwise absorbed and tends to accumulate as a poison in the bones, teeth, kidneys, thyroid, liver, brain and other vital organs, causing impairment of health. Fluoride is a major enzyme poison and fluoride accumulation is a menace to good dental health because it makes bones, teeth and connective tissue inferior and more brittle. Over time, it causes gum problems making the patient) more likely to lose his teeth.

Fluoridation - the practice of adding a high-fluoride substance to public drinking water, ostensibly for the prevention of dental caries in young children. In the past few decades, the high-fluoride substance used in the fluoridation of water comes from hazardous industrial waste, captured by the air pollution control equipment at phosphate fertilizer plants. The well-documented) health effects of water fluoridation are a sharply increased incidence of dental fluorosis, which is damage to the enamel and dentine of the tooth caused by the poisoning of the enzyme that is needed for proper collagen formation. (Collagen is the main structural protein used in the formation of teeth, bones and connective tissue.) For more information, visit the website of the Fluoride Action Network, www.FLUORIDEalert.org.

Holistore - Heavy Body Holistore is a dental composite filling material that is specially made without the addition of aluminum, iron, or other metal oxides, or) fluoride. Despite the lack of "fillers" (substance that blocks x-ray) usually used to thicken the resin, this type of Holistore is made with a heavier viscosity so that it can be used as a composite filling material.
- Holistore (light) – this is a non-toxic Holistore material made as above, but which is less viscous. This Holistore is used only for bonding crowns, inlays, onlays, or bridges onto the prepared teeth.

Homeopathy - a health care system used to treat illness and prevent disease, in which the patient is given highly diluted amounts of a substance (from a mineral, plant, or animal) in order to stimulate the body's own natural healing life-force. With the help of an expert, trained practitioner, called a homeopath, a remedy (the highly diluted substance) is chosen, from a wide range of possible remedies, to match the overall condition of the patient. Dentists trained in the use of homeopathy may use homeopathic remedies for patients wishing to alleviate pain, fight off infection and speed recovery from a surgery.

Mercury - an extremely toxic metallic element, liquid at room temperature, which has been used in thermometers, vaccine preservatives (the highly toxic and dangerous thimerosal), and dental amalgam fillings, which are about 50% mercury. The use of mercury in thermometers is being phased out. Mercury is the most poisonous metal that we are commonly exposed to. It is more poisonous than lead, cadmium or even arsenic. All unnecessary uses of mercury should be banned. (See amalgam).

Mercury vapor - liquid mercury rapidly evaporates as mercury vapor, which is the element mercury in vapor form. To some extent, mercury vapor is also released from the amalgam filling – even without any scratching or stimulation. But when an amalgam filling surface is scratched or stimulated, as with brushing the teeth or chewing food, the release of mercury vapor easily increases by ten-fold. Normally such releases of mercury vapor are not noticed, since mercury is an invisible gas that has no odor. However, Dr Roger Eichman, PhD, DDS, has created a demonstration of the release of mercury vapor from an amalgam filling using a miner's black light and a fluorescent screen, upon which the mercury vapor trail casts a shadow). (For Eichman's video, with detailed explanation, or other video demonstrations, call DAMS).

Opaque - not allowing the passage of light; not transparent. A dental material is radio-opaque if it blocks the passage of x-ray radiation. The addition of barium oxide to a composite filling is used to make a composite more radio-opaque than a tooth would be, so that the composite shows up more clearly on an x-ray.

Periosteum - the surface layer of hard connective tissue that covers the surface of a bone.

Plaque - a thin film of mucus, bacteria and other microorganisms and food residue that builds up on the surface of a tooth. Plaque is believed to form the basis for tooth decay and gum disease.

Resin - In dentistry, resin is the soft, plastic (usually petroleum based) part of a composite filling or crown/inlay/onlay material. To make the composite dental material harder and to give it the desired color, other materials ("fillers") are added into the resin; fillers may include iron oxide, barium oxide, aluminum compounds and fluoride compounds, all of which can adversely impact the health of some dental patients.

Stainless steel - a steel alloy having sufficient chromium to resist corrosion, oxidation, or rusting after exposure to liquids and air. Stainless steel is used in dentistry for making the cheapest crowns and braces. Health concerns about stainless steel dental materials center on the chromium, cobalt and nickel content – especially the nickel, which is a very toxic and allergenic (allergy-causing) element.

TOPAS test - a test to indicate the degree of bacterial or fungal infection that is present in a tooth or in the gum next to a tooth. A sample of the fluid that naturally flows out of the gum, between the tooth and the gum next to it, is placed in a tube containing test chemicals. The ensuing color change indicates the degree of bacterial infection. A second sample drop put into a second test tube indicates the level of fungal infection.

Appendix D

Glossary

Abscess -pus-filled cavity resulting from inflammation and usually caused by bacterial infection

Abutment - a tooth that supports one end of a bridge

Acupuncture - a method, originating in China, of treating disorders by inserting needles into the skin at points where the flow of energy is thought to be blocked (meridians)

Acid Radicals - toxins found deep within the body's cells and tissues

Acupuncture Points - points located on the skin that have been found to correlate to energy pathways of the body

Alloy - a metallurgical substance that is a mixture of two or more metals, or of a metal with a nonmetallic material; any mixture, amalgam, or compound of different materials

Amalgam - a material used as a filling for tooth cavities, consisting of a paste of powdered mercury, silver, and tin that quickly hardens

Amalgam Tattoo - when amalgam ions seep into the gum tissue and turn it dark blue or black

Anesthetic - a substance that reduces sensitivity to pain, relating to or producing loss of sensation in a specific area

Barium - a soft silver-white toxic chemical element used in alloys; barium is mixed with other dental filling material so that the filling will show up on x-rays

Premise Indirect (formally BelleGlass) Neutral - a lab-made dental material used for crowns, bridges, and inlays/onlays that has a frosted white appearance. This material contains no aluminum, iron oxides, fluoride or barium; it will not show up on x-rays.

Premise Indirect (formally BelleGlass) Shaded - a lab made dental material used for crowns, bridges, and inlays/onlays with shading to match the natural tooth color of a specific patient. It also contains iron oxides which will show up on x-rays.

Bio-Feedback - a machine that measures bodily functions by means of reading signals generated by acupuncture points on the body, and conveying that information to the practitioner and patient in real-time

Bonded - made to adhere in layers; chemically attached or fused together in layers (such as adhering a crown to a tooth)

Bridge - a set of one or more false teeth that act as a replacement for missing natural teeth that is bonded to a remaining tooth on each side of the missing tooth or teeth

Cadmium - a soft malleable toxic bluish-white metallic chemical element found in zinc, copper, and lead ores; the metal is used in dental amalgams; its compounds are used as pigments

Calcified – having become hardened; calcium deposits can form in areas such as the root of a tooth and killing the nerve

Capsular Antigen - a round or rod shaped substance, usually a protein, on the surface of a cell or bacterium that stimulates the production of an antibody

Cavitation - a disturbance in the mouth where teeth once existed, that has not healed properly; usually soft, mushy bone under the gum tissue or into the bone

Cavity - a hole in a tooth, caused by decay

Chelating/Chelation - to treat somebody with a chelating agent in order to remove a heavy metal, such as lead, mercury, or aluminum from the bloodstream

Composites - any dental material made up of different ingredients that fill a cavity

Computerized Electro Dermal Screening (CEDS) - a process for measuring the energy pathways of the body by conductance measurements at locations on the skin; screening the energy pathways by balancing or provoking the pathways with a stimulus

Conductance - a measure of the ability of an object to transmit energy

Cross-Checking - checking one acupuncture point with another acupuncture point to see what readings you get with each point

Crown - the visible part of a tooth, covered by enamel, or an artificial replacement for the visible part of a tooth that has decayed or been damaged

Current - the rate of flow of an electric charge through a conductor

Decalcification - the loss of calcium or calcium compounds from bone or teeth

Decay - to decompose, or cause something to decompose; a decayed tooth will become soft, crumbly, or mushy

Degeneration - the process of becoming physically, morally, or mentally worse

Dentine - the part of a tooth that is hard, contains calcium, lies underneath the enamel, and surrounds the pulp and root canals

Denture - a complete set of artificial teeth for the upper or lower jaw, attached to a plate

Detoxification - the process of removing toxic substances, or transforming them into something harmless

Disintegration - irreversible breaking into components or fragments

Dry Socket - a painful condition caused when the blood left by an extracted tooth fails to clot or the clot is dislodged

Electromagnetic Frequency - a type of energy emitted by all animate or inanimate objects, to a greater or lesser degree.

Enamel - a hard thin calcium-containing layer that covers and protects the crown of a tooth

Edentulous - without any teeth

Endodontics - the branch of dentistry that deals with diseases of the dental pulp

Energy - the capacity of a body or system to do work

Enzyme Inhibitor - a substance that binds to an enzyme to decrease a specific biochemical reaction

Erroneous Articulations - incorrect ways of doing, or thinking about something

Exponential - rapidly increasing in size

Far Infrared Saunas - a sauna that uses dry heat to help remove both chemicals and heavy metal toxins from the body

Fluoride – a chemical material found in dental materials and toothpastes

Galvanic Current - relating to or involving the direct-current electricity that is chemically generated between dissimilar metals, for example, in a battery

Gangrene - local death and decay of soft tissues of the body as a result of lack of blood to the area

Gingival Fluid - relating to the gum fluid

Gluten - a protein combination found in some cereals, breads, and pastas especially wheat

Gutta Percha - a fitted point used to fill up the root canal, the point is pushed all the way to the root's end

Heavy Body Holistore - a dental material that doesn't contain any aluminum, iron oxides, or fluoride but has a heavier viscosity (usually used for smaller fillings)

High speed drilling - High speed drilling runs at 350,000 revolutions per minute and is one of the main reasons for sensitive teeth, and dying or dead teeth. High speed drilling raises the temperature of the tooth at the point of drilling by 12 degrees centigrade. Water and air at the point of contact cannot cool the tooth.

Holistore - a dental filling material that contains no iron oxides, aluminum oxides, barium or fluoride. It does not show up on x-rays but can appear as decay, and these fillings must be checked carefully to be sure there is no decay. This material is used for small fillings and bonding inlays, onlays, crowns, and bridges

Homeopathic - a complementary disease treatment system in which a patient is given minute doses of substances (mineral, plant or animal) that in larger doses would produce symptoms of the disease itself

Hyperemic - an abnormally high level of blood in some part of the body

Iatrogenic - used to describe a symptom or illness brought on by a doctor's activity, manner, or therapy

Impacted tooth - a tooth that is wedged sideways against a barrier, usually the root of an adjoining tooth, and thus unable to break through the gum

Implants - a tooth or bone inserted surgically that is embedded in the surrounding tissue or bone (a tooth embedded in the jaw bone)

Infection - the reproduction and proliferation of microorganisms within the body, making one ill to some degree

Infra-orbital Foramen - a small opening in the bone just beneath the eye socket, close to the nose

Inlay - a filling made of a dental material that is inserted into a cavity in a tooth and cemented in position. Usually an inlay is made in a dental lab from an "impression" of the cavity space that has been made by the dentist and sent to the lab.

Intraosseous - administered by entering a bone, such as anesthetic being put into the bone

Light Body Holistore - flow able Holistore is a dental material of thinner viscosity used to bond crowns, inlays, and bridges

Linear - with an output that varies directly with the input

Lymphocytes - an important cell class in the immune system that produces antibodies to attack infected and cancerous cells, and is responsible for rejecting foreign tissue

Macroscopic - large enough to be seen and examined without the aid of magnifying equipment

Material Safety Data Sheet (MSDS) - a paper accompanying dental materials that lists the ingredients, physical/chemical characteristics, health hazard data and precautions for handling the material

Mercury - a poisonous, heavy silver-white metallic element that is liquid at room temperature and is used in thermometers, pharmaceuticals, and dental fillings. Dental amalgam is a mix of mercury, silver, tin, copper and zinc

Meridians - in acupuncture, one of the pathways in the body along which the body's energy is believed to flow and along which acupuncture points are located

Mercury vapors - fumes emitted by mercury silver amalgam fillings; the most toxic form of mercury. These fumes can be seen by using a black light, a fluorescent screen, and an extracted tooth containing a mercury silver amalgam filling.

When the filling is scraped, the fumes immediately become visible (similar to cigarette smoke coming off a cigarette)

Monomer - the liquid used in making a denture or partial, it is a small molecular chemical building block that is formed into a larger solid material

Neural Toxin - a substance that accumulates in the body that is considered to be harmful or poisonous to the nerves or nervous system

Nickel Alloy - a hard silvery-white metallic element that is resistant to corrosion and mixed with other metals to make a harder material

Ninth Space - the space in the jaw that is directly behind the wisdom tooth

Odontoblast - one of a layer of cells lining the pulp cavity of a tooth; aids in the formation of dentine

Odonton- tooth structure, in dental nomenclature

Opaque - not transparent, not allowing the passage of light; an opaque filling material will show up on x-rays

Oral Cavity - a hollow space inside the mouth

Oral Potential Meter II - an instrument to check galvanic currents in metal fillings, it measures the number of metal ion particles released per second from amalgam fillings

Partial denture - a dental plate or denture used to replace some missing teeth on the lower or upper jaw

Pathological - relating to disease or arising from disease

Pathology - any condition that is considered unhealthy or diseased (example: soft diseased bone in the jaw bone)

Periodontal Check - the use of a special instrument to check the gums or tissues surrounding the neck and root of a tooth

Periosteum - is a surface layer of hard, protective connective tissue that covers bone throughout the body, including the bony socket that holds a tooth

Preservative - a chemical that provides protection from decay, spoilage or infection

Fluorescent Screen - a special viewing screen to demonstrate mercury fumes come off a silver filling

Plaque - a film of saliva, mucus, bacteria, and food residues that build up on the surface of teeth. Plaque can cause tooth decay and gum disease

Pontic - a false tooth in a bridge

Posterior Palatine Foramen - a small hole in the back of the roof of the mouth; may be used to inject anesthetic prior to oral surgery

Proteolytic - relating to, characterized by, or promoting the breakdown of proteins or peptides into simpler molecules

Pulp stone - a calcification that occurs inside the middle of the tooth (pulp chamber) and usually, but not always, compromises the tooth

Resin - the plastic part of a composite filling. In addition to plastic resin, a composite may have "fillers" that include quartz, metal oxides, fluoride and or barium

Root canal - a dental treatment in which the diseased tissue in a root canal is removed and replaced with an inert material

Rubber dam - a thin sheet of latex rubber used to isolate a tooth or teeth and keep the area dry during a dental procedure

Silver amalgam - another name for an amalgam filling; these fillings contain a mix of mercury, silver, tin, copper and zinc

Slow-speed drilling – dental drilling using 20,000 revolutions per minute, that is kinder to the patient and tooth. See chapter 4 on Iatrogenic Effect of High Speed Drilling

Stainless steel - corrosion-resistant steel that has many domestic and industrial uses including making dental crowns and braces. Stainless steel often contains nickel, a toxic metal

Surgical – pertaining to the opening of an area with a scalpel or other instrument to clean or fix a compromised area

Systemic health – pertaining to the health of the whole body

Temporary - a material covering a tooth, once it has been prepared to make an inlay, crown, or bridge, for protection and chewing function

TOPAS Test – a test indicating the toxicity of the fluid around an implant or infected tooth

Trigeminal - relating to or involving the fifth cranial nerve, a mixed motor and sensory nerve that flows into the face and jaws

Turbulence - instability in the area where work is being done that disrupts the surrounding tooth structure

Vasoconstrictor - an agent that causes a rise in blood pressure by constricting the blood vessels; found in some local anesthetics

Volt - a unit of electric potential difference

Appendix E

References for Rescued By My Dentist

Chapter 1: New Solutions for Dentistry

1. National Geographic, Oct 1972 Quick Silver Slow Death

www.nationalgeographic.org

2. Iatrogenic Effect of High Speed Drilling by Dr. Ralph Turk, DDS

White paper presented at the 1987 American Academy of Biological Dentistry.

3. German language journal (the ZWR) Scholer (temperature change of 12 degrees C).

4. Henning and Prztak study (i.e., damage from negative pressure)

Professor Ravnik of Ljubljana, Yugoslavaia (enamel and dentine regions are disrupted decisively).

5. Dr. Boyd Haley, Root canal, peer review article.

6. Dr. George Meinig, DDS. Book: *Root Canal Cover Up Exposed*

Bion Press ISBN 0-945196-14-8

7. Price Pottenger Foundation. www.price-pottenger.org Root canals.

Chapter 2: Teeth, Jaw and Problems with Root Canal Treated Teeth

1. Computerized electro-dermal Screening.

a. *Interrelations of Odontons and Tonsils To Organs, and Tissue Systems*. By Reinhold Voll, M.D. Translated and fully revised by Harwig Schuldt, M.D., M.Sc. 1978 ISBN 3-88136-064-6

b. An *Eletrodermal Analysis of Biological Conductance*. By Vincent J. Speckhart, M.D. (H) copyright 2004 ISBN 0-9742533-0-3 E-mail: bioconductance@earthlink.net

2. Complementary Medicine and Dentistry contact: American Association of Acupuncture and Bio-Energetic Medicine 2512 Manoa Road, Honolulu, Hawaii 96822 Tel. (808)-946-2069. Fax: 808-946-0378

3. Holistore: Den-Mat. Corporation

Southern California Office,

21515 Vanowen St., #200

Canoga Park, CA 913003

Phone: 800-433-6628

4. Premise Indirect (formally BelleGlass): Kerr Lab, 1717 West Collins Ave. Orange, CA. 800-322-6666

Cook Dental Lab, owner Flint I. Cook, 10971 Clinic Road, Suring WI 54174 Phone: 920-842-2083

5. Cadmium:

a. Piscator M, Role of cadmium in carcinogenesis with special reference to cancer of the prostate. Environ Health Preps, 40: 107-120, 1981

b. Visser, AJ, Deklerk JN, The effect of dietary cadmium on prostate growth, Trans Am Assoc G-U Surg, 70: 66-68, 1979

c. Waalker MP, Rehm Coogan TP, et al, Cadmium exposure in rats and tumors of the prostate. I Cadmium in the Human Environment: Toxicity and d. Carcinogenicity, eds. GF Nordberg, L Allessio and RFM Herber, pp 390-400, Lyon: IARC

e. Webber MM, Selenium prevents the growth stimulatory effects of cadmium on the human prostatic endothelium, Biochem Biophys Res Comm, 127:871-877, 1985

f. Waalkes MP, Rehm S, Cadmium and prostate cancer, J Toxicol Environ Health, 43:251-269, 1994

g. Coogan TP, Bare RM, Waalkes MP Cadmium-induced DNA damage: Effects of zinc pretreatment, Tox Appl Pharm, 113:227-2733, 1992

Health JC, Daniel IR, Webb M., et al, Cadmium as a carcinogen, Nature, 193: 592-593, 1962

h. Kipling M.D., Waaterhouse JH, Cadmium and prostatic carcinoma, Lancet: 730-731, 1967

i. Shaikh ZA, Tang W, Protection against chronic cadmium toxicity by glycine, Toxicol 132; 2-3: 139-46, Feb, 1999

j. CSIRO Division of Energy Chemistry, NSW Ausralia, A comparative study of copper, lead, cadmium, and zinc in human sweat and blood, Sci Total
Environ, 74: 235-47, Aug. 1988

k. Pavia JM, Paier B, Zaninovich A, et al., Evidence suggesting that cadmium induces a non-thyroidal Illness syndrome in the rat, J Endocrinol 154: 113-7, 1997

Chapter 3: Oral Potential Meter II Reveals Hidden Health Problems

1. Nature 204: 625-54, 1964

2. J Oral Sur 37: 789-92, 1979

3. Arch Oral Biology 11: 931-36, 1966

4. An Electrical Potential applied to bone will cause demineralization at the positive electrode and calcification at the negative electrode.

Life Sci 3: 1276-79 1964 Parker, RB and Snyder, LM The electrical potential of dental plaque.

5. J D Res... 48: 795-98 1969 and JD Res... 52:199-205, 1973

Electrical potential of plaque.

6. Calcif Tissue Res...13: 53-62, 1963

7. Calcified Tissue of bone and teeth maintain a resting potential.

Tooth metabolism fails, JADA 83: 1078-80, 1971

8. Summers AO. etal. Mercury released from dental "silver" fillings increase the incidence of multiply resistant bacteria in the oral and intestinal normal flora. 1991 Annual meeting,
9. American Society For Microbiology. Dallas TX May 5-9, 1991 Abstract A137

10. Schriever W. and Diamond L.E. Electromotive forces and electric current caused by metallic dental fillings. J Dent Res. Vol 31(2):205-228, 1952

11. Stortebecker P., *Mercury Poisoning from Dental Amalgam –a Hazard to Human Brain*. Page 32-43, 1985. Bio-Probe, Inc. P.O. Box 608010, Orlando Fl 32860-8010

12. Los Angeles Times, Monday, April 16, 2007. When gums speak volumes: Heart disease, diabetes, strokes and other conditions may be linked to oral health.

Chapter 4: Harmful Effects of High Speed Drilling

1. www.worldhealthorganization.com increase in chronic disease; dead teeth promote disease

2. Trials with air and water-cooled turbines; change in pulp temperature. Edition of a German-language Journal (the ZWR) by Scholer 1987

3. HENNING and PRZTAK publication, 1987 Damage to pulp from negative pressure from turbine hand piece

4. Fetner, Ted; How to Minimize Pulpal Death: Endodontics (news paper article) research by Syngcuk Kim, DDS, PhD

5. Dr. Douglas L. Cook, DDS, personal loss of ten teeth from high speed drilling.

E-mail: dlcooks1@yahoo.com

6. Order "Smoking Teeth = Poison Gas" call IAOMT at 863-420-6373

7. George E. Meinig, D.D.S., F.A.C.D., *Root canal Cover-up Exposed!* Dentine under high powered microscope. Pages: 172, 174, 175, 176, 177, 179 & 180.

8. Mercury passing through rubber dam. www.IAOMT.org Safe removal of Amalgam Fillings.

9. Mercury passing through rubber dam. Dr. Phil Sukel D.D.S., in office testing with the Jerome Mercury Analyzer. Phone: 847-659-8500

10. Sherry A. Rogers, M.D., *Detoxify or Die*. Sand Key Company, Inc., Sarasota: 2002.

11. Sherry Rogers, M.D. *The High Blood Pressure Hoax*. 2005, Sand Key Company, Inc. 800-846-6687 www.prestigepublishing.com ISBN 1887202-05-6

12. Eichman: IAOMT seminar, Huston Texas, 2001

Chapter 5: Dental Office Location - A Practice Management Concern

1. Morley Safer: 60 Minutes NBC 12/16/90 Is There Poison in Your Teeth?

2. Clarkson T. Metal toxicity in the central nervous system. Environmental Health Perspect. 1987; 75:59-64.

3. Friberg Lars, Mordberg GF, Gunner F, Vouk VB, Velmir B, eds. Handbook on the Toxicology of Metals. Vol I New York, NY: Elservier Science Publishing Co; 1986.

4. Martell A#. Chemistry of carcinogenic metals. Environ Health Perspect. 1981; 40:207-226.

5. Stortebecker P. The cranial venous system filled from the pulp of a tooth. Proceedings of the Third International Congress of Neurological Surgery, Copenhagen, Denmark, August 1965. Pp. 635-636.

6. Stortebecker P. Dental caries as a cause of nervous disorders. Stockholm, Sweden: Foundation for Research; 1982.

7. Cutright DE, Miller RA, Battistone GC, Milikan LJ. Systemic mercury levels caused by inhaling mist during high speed amalgam grinding. J Oral Med. 1973; 28:100-104.

8. Svare CW, Peterson LC, Reinhaart JW, et al. The effect of dental amalgams on mercury levels in expired air. J Dental Res. 1981; 60:1668-1671.

9. Wranglen G, Bevendson J. Electrochemical aspects of corrosion processes in the oral cavity with special reference to amalgam fillings. Corrosion and Surface Protection of Metals. Stockholm, Sweden: Royal Institute of Technology, 1983.

10. National Geographic 1972. October issue: "Quick Silver Slow Death."

11. Andreas Moritz, *The Amazing Liver and Gallbladder* Flush, 2007

12. F. Batmanghelidj, M.D. *Your Body's Many Cries for Water*, 1992

Chapter 6: Dental Health Begins One Step At A Time

1. *Detoxify Or Die* by Sherry A. Rogers, M.D. 2002 1-800-486-6687 www.prestigepublishing.com

2. *You Are What You Ate* (Revised) Sherry A. Rogers, M.D. Third Edition Second Printing 2000 www.prestigepublishing.com

3. *The Body Ecology Diet* by Donna Gates 1996 call 800-511-2660 www.bodyecologydiet.com

4. *Gut and Psychology Syndrome (Natural Treatment for Dyspraxia, Autism, A.D.H.D, Depression, Schizophrenia* by Dr. Natasha Campbell-McBride M.D. Seventh printing 2007 800-511-2660

5. *The High Blood Pressure Hoax!* by Sherry A. Rogers, M.D. 2005 1-800-486-6687 www.prestigepublishing.com

6. *Obesity Cancer Depression* by F. Batmanghelidj, M.D. 2004 Global Health Solutions Tel. 703-848-2333 www.watercure.com

7. *ABC of Asthma, Allergies, & Lupus* by F. Batmanghelidj, M.D. 2000 Global Health Solutions Tel. 703-848-2333 www.watercure.com

8. *Your Body's Many Cries for Water* by F. Batmanghelidj, M.D. 1997 Global Health Solutions Tel. 703-848-2333 www.watercure.com

9. Webb M, Clinical Chemistry and Chemical Toxicology of Metals. S. Brown, ed. Amsterdam, The Netherlands: Elsevier; 1977:51-64.

10. Swartzendruber DE. Adverse immunomodulatory effects of heavy metals in dental materials. Proceedings from the International Conference on Biocompatibility of Materials, 1988

11. Magos L., Mercury-blood interaction and mercury uptake by the brain after vapor exposure. Environ Res. 1967; 1:323-327.

12. CRIRO Division of Energy Chemistry, NSW Australia, A comparative study of copper, lead, cadmium and zinc in human sweat and blood, Sci Total Environ,74:235-47 Aug 1988

13. Pavia JM, Paier B, Zaninovich A, et al, Evidence suggesting that cadmium induces a non-thyroidal illness syndrome in the rat, J Endocrinol 154:113-7, 1997

14. Waalkes MP, Rehm S, Cadmium and prostate cancer, J Toxicol Environ Health, 42:251-269, 1994

15. Shaikkh ZA, Tang W, Protection against chronic cadmium toxicity by glycine, Toxicol 132; 2-3: 139-46, Feb 151,999

16. Sherry Rogers, M.D. *The Cholesterol Hoax* 2008 by Sand Key Company, Inc. 800-846-6687 ISBN: 978-1-887202-06-0

Chapter 7: Computerized Electro-dermal Screening: What Patients and Dentists Need to Know

1. Computerized Electro-dermal Screening.

a. *Interrelations of Odontons and Tonsils To Organs, and Tissue Systems*. By Reinhold Voll, M.D. Translated and fully revised by Harwig Schuldt, M.D.,M.Sc. 1978 ISBN 3-88136-064-6

b. *An Eletrodermal Analysis of Biological Conductance*. By Vincent J. Speckhart, M.D. (H) copyright 2004 ISBN 0-9742533-0-3 E-mail irders: bioconductance@earthlink.net

2. American Association of Acupuncture and Bio-Energetic Medicine 2512 Manoa Road, Honolulu, Hawaii 96822 Tel. (808)-946-2069. Fax: 808-946-0378

3. *Body Electric* by Roberts Becker

4. *Cross Currents* by Robert Becker

Chapter 8: All Metals Carry Electrical Current, No Metals Are Not Compatible

1. Clarke, A. *Dictionary of Practical Materia Medica* by John Henry Clarke Published by B. Jain Publishers (P) LTD. Aurum metallicum (gold) pages 224-227. Reprint Edition: 1993 ISBN 81-7021-0190-4 and ISBN 81-7021-013-5

2. *Materia Medica with Repertory* by William Boericke, M.D. with the addition of a Repertory by Oscar E. Boericke, A.B., M.D. June 1927

3. Konetzka W. Microbiology of metal transformation. In Weinberg, ED, ed. Micro-organism and Minerals. New York, NY; Mark Dekker, Inc.; 1977:317-342

4. Sterzl I, et al, Mercury and nickel allergy: risk factors in fatigue and auto-immunity, Neruoendocrinology Letters 20: 221-28, 1999.

Loken, A.C., Lung cancer in nickel workers. Tidsskr NorLaegeferen 70:376, 1950

5. Fursi, A., Haro, R.T., and Schlauder, M: Experimental chemotherapy of nickel induced fibro-sarcomas. Oncology 26:422, 1972

6. Gilman, J.P.W.: Metal carcinogenesis II W study of the carcinogenic activity of cobalt, copper, iron, and nickel compounds. Cancer Res 22:158, 1962.

7. Clarke, Materia Medica Niccolum (nickel) Page 580-584 symptoms: low spirited, fears something evil will happen, anxiety. Dullness, does not comprehend the conversation, headaches. Etc.

8. Clarke, *Materia Medica* Reprint Edition: 1993 page. 224-229 Aurum Metallicum (Gold) Mind. Melancholy, suicidal. Head-vertigo and etc.

9. TF Bladet Issue # 1 2008 Implant - allergy to titanium (In Swedish)

Chapter 9: Root Canal Treatments ("Root canals") May Adversely Affect Your Health

1. Waalkes MP, Rehm S, Cadmium and prostate cancer, J Toxicol Environ Health, 43:251-269,1994

2. Coogan TP, Bare RM, Waalker MP, Cadmium-induced DNA damage: Effects of zinc pretreatment, Tox Appl Pharm, 113:227-233, 1992

Heath JC, Daniel IR, Webb M., et al, Cadmium as a carcinogen, Nature, 193:592-593, 1962

3. Refer to Dr. Volls Book: *Interrelations of Odontons And Tonsils To Organs, Fields Of Disturbance, And Tissue Systems*. 1978 ISBN 3-88136-064-6 Gesamtherstellung: C.Geckers Buchdruckeri BmbH & Co. KG., D-3110 Uelzen 1

4. Root Canal Cover Up Exposed by Dr. George Meinig, DDS,

Weston Price's work on root canals is found at Price Pottinger foundation, www.price-pottenger.org.

5. Dental Infections and Oral and Systemic vol. 1 1923 Weston A. Price, D.D.S., M.S., F.A.C.D.

6. Research On Clinical Expressions of Dental Infections vol. 2 1923 Weston A. Price, D.D.S., M.S., F.A.C.D.

7. Mouth infections and a review of the literature Vol.1 and Vol. 2 by Malcolm Graeme MacNevin, M.D., F.A.C.P. and Harol Stearns Vaughan, M.D., D.D.S., F.A.C.S.

8. Dental infections foci and diseases of the nervous system by Tore Patrick Stortebecker Oslo, Norway 1961

9. Nair, P, Sjogren, U, Krey, G, Kahnberg, KE, Sundqvist, G. Intraradicular bacteria and fungi in root-filled, asymptomatic human teeth with therapy-resistant periapical lesions; a long-term light and electron microscopic follow-up study. Dental Institute, University of Zurich, Switzerland. J.Endod 1990 Dec: 16(12):580-588.

10. Perez F, Calas P, de Falguerolles A, Maurette, A. Migration of a streptococcus sanguis strain through the root dentinal tubules.

11. Service d'Odontologie Conseratrice-Endodontie, Faculte De Chirurgie Dentaire, Toulouse, France. J endod 1993 June, 19(6):297-301.

12. Ando M, Hoshoio E. Predominant obligate anaerobes invading the deep layers of root canal dentin. Department of Oral Microbiology, School of Dentistry, Niigata University, Japan, Int Endod J 1990 Jan; 23(1): 20-27.

Giuliana G, Ammatuna P, Pizo G, Capone F, and D'Angelo M., Occurrence of invading bacteria in ridiculer dentin of periodontally diseased teeth: microbiological findings.

13. Department of Periodontology, University of Palermo, Italy.

J Clin Periodontol 1997 Jul; 24(7): 478-485.

14. Kerekes, K, Olsen, I. Similarities in the microfloras of root canals and deep periodontal pockets. Dental Faculty, University of Oslo, Norway. Eneod Dent Rraumatol 1990 Feb; 6(1):1-5.

15. Kobayashi T, Hayashi A, Yoshikawa R, Okuda K, Hara K, The microbial flora from root canals and periodontal pockets of non-vital teeth associated with advanced periodontitis. Niigata University School of Dentistry, Japan. Int Endod J 1990 Mar; 23(2):100-106.

16. Liang JP, [Anaerobes in infected canals: a preliminary study.]

[article in Chiniese] College of Stomatology, Shanghai Second Medical University. Chung Hua Kou Chiang Hsueh Tsa Chih 1991 Jan; 26(1):28-30.

Baumgartner JC, Falkler WA JR, Bacteria in the apical 5mm of infected root canals.

17. Microbiology Branch United State Army Institute of Dental Research Walter Reed Army Medical Center, Washington, DC.

J Endod 1991 Aug; 17(8):380-383.

18. Hirai K, Tagami A, Okuda K, Isolation and classification of anaerobic bacteria from pulp cavities of nonvital teeth in man.

Tokyo Dental College. Bull Tokyo Dent Coll Aug; 32(3): 95-98.

19. Kipioti A, Makou M, Legakis N, Mitsis F, Microbiological findings of infected root canals and adjacent periodontal pockets in teeth with advanced periodontitis.

20. Oral Surg Oral Med Oral Pathol 1984 Aug; 58(2):231-220.

Ogunebi BR, Dentin tubule infection and endodontic therapy implications.

Department of endodontics, University of Florida, College of Dentistry, Gainesville 32610-0436

Int Endod J 1994 Jul; 27 (4):218-222.

21. Ueno K, Yoshihashi M, Sawada N, Nakajima M, Araki K, Suda K, [Cytotoxicity of anaerobic bacteria isolated from infected root canal]. Department of Endodontics, Faculty of Dentistry, Tokyo Medical and Dental University

Infect Immun 1986 Jul; 53(1):149-153.

22. Haapasalo M, Ranta H, Ranta K, Shah H, Black-pigmented Bacteroides spp. In human apical periodontitis.

Infect Immun 1986 Jul; 53(1):149-153.

23. Preda EG, Pasetti P, [Focal pathology and infectious dental foci. Theoretical and clinical aspects].

Universita Digli Studi di Pavia. Dent Cadmos 1990 Jul 15; 58(12):34-43.

Gomes BP, Lilley JD, Drucker DB

24. Clinical significance of dental root canal microflora. Restorative Dentistry, University Dental Hospital of Manchester, UK. J Dent 1996 Jan; 24(1-2):47-55.

25. Taniguchi N, Fujisawa M, Shinohara K, Uetani T, Tadano H, Horiguchi H, Sekine I, [Research on aseptic condition of root canals after endodontic treatment].

Oral Microbiol Immunol 1992 Oct; 7(5): 257-262.

26. Molven O, Olsen I, Kerekes, K, Scanning electron microscopy of bacteria in the apical part of the root canals in permanent teeth with periapical lesions.

Endod Dent Traumatol 1991 Oct; 7(5):226-229.

27. Debelian GJ, Olsen I, Tronstad L, Electrophoresis of whole-cell soluble proteins of microorganisms isolated from bacteremias in endodontic therapy.

Department of Oral Biology, University of Oslo, Norway. gilbert@odonto.unio.no

Eur J Oral Sci 1996 Oct; 104(5-6):540-546

28. Debelian GJ, Olsen I, Tronstad L, Bacteremia in conjunction with endodontic therapy.

Division of Endodontics, Department of Oral Biology, Faculty of Dentistry, University of Oslo, Norway

Endod Dent Traumatol 1995 Jun; 11(3):142-149

29. Giuliana G, Ammatuna P, Pizzo G, Capone F, D'Angelo M, Occurrence of invading bacteria in radicular dentin of periodontally diseased teeth: microbiological findings.

Department of Periodontology, University of Palermo, Italy

J Clin Periodontol 1997 Jul; 24(7):478-485

30. Kerekes, K, Olsen I, Similarities in the microfloras of root canals and deep periodontal pockets.

Dental Faculty, University of oslo, Norway

Endod Dent Traumatol 1990 Feb; 6(1):1-5

31. Kobayashi T, Hayashi A, Yoshikawa R, Okuda K, Hara K, The microbial flora from root canals and periodontal pockets of non-vital teeth associated with advanced periodontitis.

Niigata University School of Dentistry, Japan

Int Endod J 1990 Mar: 23(2):100-106

32. Kipioti A, Nakou M, Legakis N, Mitsis F, Microbiological findings of infected root canals and adjacent periodontal pockets in teeth with advanced periodontitis.

Oral Surg Oral Med Oral Pathol 1984 Aug; 58(2):213-220

33. Gharbia SE, Haapasalo M, Shah HN, Kotiranta A, Lounatmaa K, Pearce MA, Devine DA, Characterization of Prevotella intermedia and Prevotella nigrescens isolates from periodontic and endodontic infections.

Faculty of Dentistry, Dalhousie University, Halifax, Nova Scotia, and J Periodontol 1994 Jan; 65(1):56-61

34. Ando N, Hoshino E, Sato M, Kota K, Iwaku M, Culture conditions for efficient recovery of bacteria from infected dental root canals.

Shika Kiso Igakkai Zasshi 1989 Oct. 31(5):603-608

35. Liang JP [Anaerobes in infected canals: a preliminary study].

College of Stomatology, Shanghai Second Medical University

Chung Hua Kou Chiang Hsueh Tsa Chih 1991 Jan; 26(1):28-30

36. Baumgartner JC, Falkler WA Jr., Bacteria in the apical 5 mm of infected root canals. Microbiology Branch, United States Army Institute of Dental Research, Walter Reed Army Medical Center, Washington, DC.

J Endod 1991 Aug; 17(8):380-383

37. Hirai K, Tagami A, Okuda K, Isolation and classification of anaerobic bacteria from pulp cavities of nonvital teeth in man.

Tokyo Dental College

Bull Tokyo Dent Coll 1991 Aug; 32(3):95-98

38. Nair P, Sjogren U, Krey G, Kahnberrg KE, Sundqvist G, Intraradicular bacteria and fungi in root-filled, asymptomatic human

teeth with therapy-resistant periapical lesions: a long-term light and electron microscopic follow-up study.

Dental Institute, University of Zurich, Switzerland

J. Endod 1990 Dec; 6(12):580-588

39. Perez F, Calas P, de Falguerolles A, Maurette A, Migration of a Streptococcus sanguis strain through the root dentinal tubules.

Service d'Odontologie Consercatrice-Endodontie, Faculte de Chirurgie Dentaire, Toulouse, France

J Endod 1993 jun; 19(6):297-301

40. Ando N, Hoshino E, Predominant obligate anaerobes invading the deep layers of root canal dentin.

Department of Oral Microbiology, School of Dentistry, Niigata University, Japan

Int Endod J 1990 Jan; 23(1):20-27

41. Chaou WS, Turng BF, Minah GE, Coll JA, Inhibition of pure cultures of oral bacteria by root canal filling materials.

Department of Microbiology, University of Maryland Dental School, Baltimore, USA

Pediatr Sent 1996 Nov; 18(7):444-449

42. Moritz A, Doertbudak O, Gutknecht N, Goharkhay K, Schoop U Sperr W, Nd: YAG laser irradiation of infected root canals in combination with microbiological examinations.

Department of Conservative Dentistry, Dental School, University of Vienna, Wien, Austria

J Am Dent Assoc 1997 Nov. 128(11):525-1530

43. Klinke T, Klimm W, Gutknecht N, Antibacterial effects of Nd: YAG laser irradiation within root canal dentin.

Outpatients" Department of Operative Dentistry and Periodontics of the Center of Dentistry, University Clinical Center Carl Gustav Carus, Dresden Technical University, Germany.

J Clin Laser Med Surg 1997 Feb; 15(1):29-31

44. Kontakiotis E, Nakou M, Georgopoulou M, In vitro study of the indirect action of calcium hydroxide on the anaerobic flora of the root canal.

Department of Endodontics, Dental School, Athens, Greece

Int Endod J 1995 Nov; 28(6):285-289

45. Siqueira Junior JF, Uzeda M, Disinfection by calcium hydroxide pastes of dentinal tubules infected with two obligate and one facultative anaerobic bacteria.

Oral Microbiology Laboratory, Institute of Microbiology, Federal University of Rio De Janeiro, Brazil

46. Georgopoulou M, Kontakiotis E, Nakou M, In vitro evaluation of effectiveness of calcium hydroxide and paramonochlorophenol from the root canal.
Department of Endodontics, Dental School, Athens, Greece

Endod Dent Traumatol 1993 Dec; 9(6):249-253

47. Fukushima H, Yamamotto K, Hirohata K, Sagawa H, Leung KP, Walker CB, Localization and identification of root canal bacteria in clinically asymptomatic periapical pathosis.

College of Dentistry, University of Florida, Gainesville

J Endod 1990 Nov; 16(11):534-538

48. Debelian GJ, Olsen I, Tronstad L, Profiling of Propionibacteruim acnes recovered from root canal and blood during and after endodontic treatment.

Division of Endodontics, University of Oslo, Norway

Endod Dent Traumatol 1992 Dec; 8(6):248-254

49. Sundqvist G, Johansson E, Sjogren U, Prevalence of black-pigmented bacteroides species in root canal infections.

J Endod 1889 Jan; 15(1):13-19

50. Haapasalo M, Black-pigmented gram-negative anaerobes in endodontic infections.

Department of Cariology, University of Helsinki, Finland

FEMS Immunol Med Microbiol 1993 Mar; 6(2-3):213-217

51. Haapasalo M, Bacteroides buccae and related taxa in necrotic root canal infections.

J Clin Microbial 1986 Dec; 24(6):940-944

56. Sundqvist G, Associations between microbial species in dental root canal infections.

University of Umea, Sweden

Oral Microbiol Immunol 1992 Oct; 7(5):257-262

57. Chaudhry R, Kalra N, Talwar V, Thakur R, Anaerobic flora in endodontic infections.

Department of Microbiology, University College of Medical Sciences, Delhi

Indian J Med Res 1997 Jun; 105:262-265

58. Kerosuo E, Haapasalo M, Lounatmaa K, Ranta H, Ranta K, Ultrastructure of a novel anaerobic gram-positive nonsporing rod from dental root canal.

Department of Cariology, University of Helsinki, Finland

Scand J Dent Res 1988 Feb; 96(1):50-55

59. Drucker DB, Lilley JD, Tucker D, Gibbs AC, The endodontic microflora revisited.

Department of Cell and Structural Biology, Turner Dental School, University Manchester, Great Britain

Microbios 1992; 71(288-289):225-234

60. Ehnevid H, Jansson L, lindskog S, Weintraub A, Blomiof L, Endodontic pathogens: propagation of infection through patent dentinal tubules in traumatized monkey teeth

Department of Oral History and Cell Biology, Karolinska Institutet, Stochholm, Sweden

Endod Dent Traumatol 1995 Oct; 11(5):229-234

61. Le Goff A, Bunetel L, Mouton C, Bonnaure-Mallet M, Evaluation of root canal bacteria and their antimicrobial susceptibility in teeth with necrotic Pulu

Equipe de Biologie Buccal, Faculte d'Odontologie, Universite de Renna, France

Oral Microbiol Immunoln1997 Oct; 12(5):318-322

62. Dahle UR, Tronstad L, Olsen I, Spirochetes in oral infection

Division of Endodontics, University of Oslo, Norway

Endod Dent Traumatol 1993 Jun; 9(3):87-94

63. Dahle UR, Tronstad L, Olsen I, Observation of an unusually large spirochete in endodontic infection

Division of Endodontics and Department of Microbiology, Dental Faculty, University of Olso, Norway

Oral Microbiol Immunol 1993 Aug; 8(4):251-253

64. Haapasalo M, Bacteroides spp. In dental root canal infection

Endod Dent Traummatol 1989 Feb; 5(1):1-10

65. Debelian GJ, Olsen I, Tronstad L, Systemic diseases caused by oral micro-organisms

Division of Endodontics, University of Oslo, Norway

Endod Dent Traumatol 1994 Apr; 10(2):57-65

66. Navszesh M, Mulligan R, Systemic dissemination as a result of oral infection in individuals 50 years of age and older

Department of Dental Medicine & Public Health, University of Southern California, School of Dentistry, Los Angeles 90089-0641, USA

Spec Care Dentist 1995 Jan; 15(1):11-19

67. Debelian GJ, Olsen I, Tronstad L, Electrophoresis of whole-cell soluble proteins of microorganisms isolated from bacteremias in endodontic therapy

Department of Oral Biology, University of Oslo, Norway, gilbert@odont.uio.no

Eur J Oral Sci 1996 Oct; 104(5-6):540-546

68. Debelian GJ, Olsen I, Tronstad L, Bacteremia in conjunction with endodontic therapy

Division of Endodontics, Department of Oral Biology, Faculty of Dentistry, University of Olso, Norway

Endod Dent Traumatol 1995 Jun; 11(3):142-149

Chapter 10: Replacing Missing Teeth

1. TOPAS Test: ALT BioScience 235 Bolivar Street Lexington, KY 40508 phone 859-388-9445

2. Computerized Electro-dermal Screening: Check energy of implant material against the energy of the patient.

3. Heath JC, Daniel IR, Webb M., et al, Cadmium as a carcinogen, Nature, 193:592-593, 1962

4. Waalkes MP, Rehm S, Cadmium and prostate cancer, J Toxicol Environ Health, 43:251-269,1994

5. Coogan TP, Bare RM, Waalker MP, Cadmium-induced DNA damage: Effects of zinc pretreatment, Tox Appl Pharm, 113:227-233, 1992

Chapter 11: Fluoride A Neurotoxin

1. References: *Fluoride the Aging Factor* by Dr. John Yiamonuyiannis ISBN 0-913571-01-6

2. A. Benagiano, The effect of sodium fluoride on thyroid enzymes and basal metabolism in the rat, Annali Di Stomatologia, Volume 13 pp. 601-619 (1965)

V. Stolc and J. Podoba, Effect of fluoride on the biogenesis of thyroid hormones, Nature, Volume 188, No. 4753, pp. 855-856 (1960).

3. *Detoxify or Die*, by Sherry Rogers, M.D. Fluoride, pages 19, 21, 22

4. Paul Connett, Why water fluoridation must be ended, Dental Truth Fall 2007 winter 2008 (published February 2008) phone: 800-311-6265 Leo Cashman contact person

Chapter 12: Tooth and Jaw Case Histories

1. Refer to Dr. Volls Book: *Interrelations of Odontons And Tonsils To Organs, Fields Of Disturbance, And Tissue Systems*. 1978 ISBN 3-88136-064-6 Gesamtherstellung: C.Geckers Buchdruckeri BmbH & Co. KG., D-3110 Uelzen 1

2. Dr. George Meinig is the author of *Root Canal Cover Up Exposed.*

3. Dr. Boyd Haley, is a professor of Chemistry and Toxicologist at the University of Kentucky

Chapter 13: The Oral Cavity: A Cause of Health Problems

1. In Review of NICO *Neuralgia-inducing Cavitational Osteonecrosis, G.V. Black's Forgotten Disease* 4th edition; 1995

2. J.E. Bouquot, D.D.S., M.S.D. Director of Research, The Maxillofacial Center for Diagnostics & Research, Director, Head & Neck Diagnostics of America, Visiting Senior Scientist, Mayo clinic, Rochester, Minnesota

3. Complete Listing of NICO Publications (by date of publication):

4. Black G.V., A *Work on Special Dental Pathology*. Chicago, Medico-Dental Publ Co, 1915

5. Adler E., *Neural Social Dentistry*. Huston, TX, Multi-discipline Research Foundation, 1984 (1st German ed. =1976)

6. Ratner EJ, Person P, Kleinman DJ. Oral pathology and trigeminal neuralgia. I. Clinical experiences. J Dent Res 1976; 55:299. (abstr)

7. Shklar G, Person P, Ratner E. Oral pathology and trigeminal neuralgia. II Histopathologic observations. J Dent Res 1976; 55(B): 299. (abstr)

8. Socransky SS, Stone C, Ratner E. Oral pathology and trigeminal neruralgia. III Microbiologic examination. J Dent Res 1976; 55(B): 300. (abstr)

9. Ratner EJ, PersonP, Kleinman DJ., Severe arm pain associated with pathological bone cavity of maxilla. Lancet 1978: 106-107

10. Ratner EJ, Person P, Kleinman DJ, et al. Jawbone cavities and trigeminal and atypical facial neuralgias. Oral Surg. 1979; 48:3-20.

11. Roberts AM, Person P. Etiology and treatment of idiopathic trigeminal and atypical facial neuralgias. Oral Surg 1979; 48:298-308.

12. Shaber EP, Krol AJ. Trigeminal neuralgia--a new treatment concept. Oral Surg 1980; 49:286-293, 1980.

13. Mathis BJ, Oatis GW, Grisius RJ. Jaw Bone cavities associated with facial pain syndromes: case reports. Milit Med 1981: 146:719-723.

14. Jiao X, Meng Q. [The influence of pathologic bone cavity of jaw bone on the etiopathology of trigeminal neuralgia.] Acta Acd Med Sichuan 1981; 243-247.

15. Wang M, Xiwei J, Qingrong I, sanyou Z. [A study of the relation between the various trigger zones of idiopathic trigeminal neuralgia and jaw bone cavities.] Acta Acad Med Sichuan 1982; 13:233-238.

16. Wang M, Xiwei J, Meng Q, etal. [Localization method in the diagnosis of the pathological jaw bone cavity.] Acta Acad Med Sichuan 1982; 13:341-344.

17. Demerath RR, Sist T. Treatment of osteocavitition lesions in facial pain patients: preliminary results. J Dent Res 1982; 61:218. (abstr)

18. Grecko VE, Puzin MN. [Odontogenic trigeminal neuralgia] Zh Nevropathol Psikhiatr 1984; 84(11): 1655-1658.

19. Roberts AM, Person P, Chandran NB; 58:121-129.

20. Ratner EJ, Langer B, Evins ML. Alverolar cavitational ostepathosis--manifestations of an infectious process and its implication in the causation of chronic pain. J Periodontol 1986: 57:593-603.

21. Bouquot JE, Roberts AM, Person, P, Christian J, The histopathology of neuralgia-inducing cavitational osteonecrosis (NICO). J Dent Res 1989; 68:952. (abstr)

22. Bouquot J, Christian J. Long-term effects of jawbone curettage on the pain of facial neuralgia; treatment results in neuralgia-inducing cavitational osteonecrosis. Oral Surg 1991: 72:582. (abstr)

23. Segall RO, Del Rio CE. Cavitational bone defect: a diagnostic challenge. J Endo 1991; 17:396-400.

24. McMahon RE, Griep J, Marfurt CP. Local anesthetic effects in the presence of chronic osteomyelitis of the mandible. Anesth Prog 1991; 38:189.

25. McMahon RE, Griep J, Marfurt CP. Local anesthetic effects in the presence of chronic osteomyelitis of the mandible. J Orofacial Pain 1992; 7:116. (abst)

26. Bouquot JE, Roberts AM, Person P, Christian J. NICO (neuralgia-inducing cavitational osteonecrosis): oateomyelitis in 224 jawbone samples from patients with facial neuralgias. Oral Surg 1992; 73:307-319.

27. Donlon WC. Invited commentary on neuralgia-inducing cavitational osteonecrosis. Oral Surg 1992; 73:319-320.

28. Bouquot JE. More on the neuralgia-inducing cavitational osteonecrosis (NICO). Oral Surg 1992; 74:348-350.

29. McMahon RE, Adams W, Spolnik K. Diagnostic anesthesia for referred trigeminal pain, parts I 7 II Compendium Cont Educ Dent 1992; 11:870-881, 980-997.

30. Carlsson, J., Larsen, J.T., and Edlund, M.-B. (1993). Peptostreptococcus micros have a uniquely high capacity to form hydrogen sulfide from glutathione. Oral Microbiol. Immunol. 8, 42-45.

31. Debelian, G.J., Olsen, I., and Tronstad, L. (1994). Systemic diseases caused by oral microorganisms.

Endod. Dent. Traumatol. 10, 57-65

32. De Boever, E.H., De Uzeda, M., and Loesche, W.J. (1994). Relationship between volatile sulfur compounds, BANA-hydrolyzing bacteria and gingival health in patients with and without complaints of oral malodor. J. Clin. Dent. 4, 114-119.

33. Nord CE, Heimdahl A, Cardiovascular Infections: bacterial endocarditis of oral origin. Pathogenesis and prophylaxis.

Department of Microbiology, Huddinge University Hospital, Karolinska Institute, Stockholm, Sweden

J Clin Periodontol 1990 Aug: 17(7 Pt 2):494-496

34. Verhaaren H, Claeys G, Verschraegen G, de Niel C, Leroy J, Clement D, Endocarditis from a dental focus. Importance of oral hygiene in valvar heart disease.

Department of Pediatrics, University Hospital, Gent State University, Belgium.

Int J Cardiol 1989 Jun; 23(3):343-347

35. Grau AJ, Buggle F, Zielgler C, Schwarz W, Meuser J, Tasman AJ, Buhler A, Benesch C, Becher H, Hacke W, Association between acute cerebrovascular ischemia and chronic and recurrent infection.

Department of Neurology, University of Heidelberg, Germany.

Stroke 1997 Sep; 28(9):1724-1729

36. Syrjanen J, Peltola J, Valtonen V, Iivanainen M, Kaste M, Huttunen JK, Dental infections in association with cerebral infarction in young and middle-aged men.

Department in Bacteriology and Immunology, University of Helsinki, Finland.

J Intern Med 1989 Mar; 225(3):179-184

37. Mattila KJ, Valle MS, Nieminen MS, Valtonen VV, Hietaniemi KL, Dental infections and coronary atherosclerosis.

First Department of Medicine, Helsinki University Central Hospital, Finland

Atherosclerosis 1993 Nov; 103(2):205-211

38. Beck J, Garcia R, Heiss G, Vokonas PS, Offenbacher S, Periodontal disease and cardiovascular disease.

Department of Dental Ecology, University of North Carolina, Chapel Hill, USA

J. Periodontal 1996 Oct; 67(10 Suppl):1123-1137

39. Loesche WJ, Periodontal disease as a risk factor for heart disease.

School of Medicine, University of Michigan, Ann Arbor

Compendium 1994 Aug; 15(8):976

40. Duhr EF, Pendergrass JC, Stevin JT, Haley BE, Hg EDTA complex inhibits GTP interactions with the E-site of brain beta-tubulin.

41. Division of Medicinal Chemistry and Pharmaceutical, College of Pharmacy, University of Kentucky Medical Center, Lexington

Toxicol Appl Pharmacol 1993 Oct; 122(2):273-280

42. Pendergrass JC, Haley BE, Vimy MJ, Winfield SA, Lorscheider FL, Mercury vapor inhalation inhibits binding of GTP to tubulin in rat brain: similarity to a molecular lesion in Alzheimer diseased brain.

College of Pharmacy, University of Kentucky, Lexington 40536, USA

Neurotoxicology 1997; 18(2):315-324

43. Pendergrass JC, Haley BE, Inhibition of brain tubulin-guanosine 5'-triphosphate interactions by mercury: similarity to observations in Alzheimer diseased brain.

College of Pharmacy, Division of Medicinal Chemistry and Pharmaceutics, University of Kentucky Medical Center, Lexington 40536-0082, USA

Met Ions Biol Syst 1997; 34:461-478

44. Hayden LJ, Goeden H, Roth SH, Growth and development in the rat during sub-chronic exposure to low levels of hydrogen sulfide.

Department of Pharmacology and Therapeutics, University of Calgary, Alberta, Canada

Toxicol Ind Health 1990May; 6(3-4):389-401

45. Hayden LJ, Goeden H, Roth SH, Exposure to low levels of hydrogen sulfide elevates circulating glucose in maternal rats.

Department of Pharmacology and Therapeutics, University of Calgary, Alberta, Canada

J Toxicol Environ Health 1990 Sep; 31(1):45-52

46. Kangas J, Jappinen P, Savolainen H, Exposure to hydrogen sulfide, mercaptans and sulfur dioxide in pulp industry.
Am Ind Hyg Assoc J 1984 Dec; 45(12):787-790

47. Pitcher MC, Cummings JH, Hydrogen sulfide: a bacterial toxin in ulcerative colitis?

MRC Dunn Clinical Nutrition Centre, Cambridge

Gut 1996 Jul; 39(1):1-4

48. Reiffenstein RJ, Hulbert WC, Roth SH, Toxicology of hydrogen sulfide.

Department of Pharmacology, University of Alberta, Edmonton, Canada

Annu Rev Pharmacology Toxicol 1992; 32:109-134

49. Guidotti TL, Hydrogen sulfide.

Occupational Health Program, University of Alberta, Faculty of Medicine, Edmonton, Canada

Occup Med (Oxf) 1996 Oct; 46(5):367-371

50. Khan AA, Yong S, Prior MG, Lillie LE, Cytotoxic effects of hydrogen sulfide on pulmonary alveolar macrophages in rats.

Animal Sciences Division, Alberta Environmental Centre, Vegreville, Canada

J Toxicol Environ Health 1991 May; 33(1):57-64

51. Pianotti R, Lachette S, Dillis S, Desulfuration of cysteine and methionine by Fusobacterium nucleatum

J Dent Res 1986 Jun; 65(6):913-917

52. Tansy MF, Kendall FM, Fantasia J, Landin WE, Oberly R, Sherman W, Acute and sub chronic toxicity studies of rats exposed to vapors of methyl mercaptan and other reduced-sulfur compounds

J Toxicol Environ Health 1981 Jul; 8(1-2); 71-88

53. J Johnson PW, Ng W, Tonzetich J, Modulation of human gingival fibroblast cell metabolism by methyl mercaptan

Department of Oral Biology, Faculty of Dentistry, University of British Columbia, Vancouver, Canada

J Periodontal Res 1992 Sep; 27(5):476-483

54. Waler SM, On the transformation of sulfur-containing amino acids and peptides to volatile sulfur compounds (VSC) in the human mouth.

Dental Faculty, University of Oslo, Norway. smw@odont.uio.no

Eur J Oral Sci 1997 Oct; 105(5 Pt 2); 534-537

55. Ahmed K, Zieve L, Quarfoth G, Effects of methanethiol on erythrocyte membrane stabilization and on Na+, K+-adenosine triphosphatase: relevance to hepatic coma

J Pharmacol Exp Ther 1984 Jan; 228(1); 103-108

56. Tang-Larsen J, Claesson R, Edlund MB, Carlsson J, Competition for peptides and amino acids among periodontal bacteria

Department of Oral Microbiology, University of Umea, Sweden

J Periodontal Res 1995 Nov; 30(6):390-395

57. Roth SH, Skrajny B, Reiffenstein R, Alteration of the morphology and neurochemistry of the developing mammalian nervous system by hydrogen sulfide

Department of Pharmacology and Therapeutics, Faculty of Medicine, University of Calgary, Alberta, Canada

Clin Exp Pharmacol Physical 1995 May; 22(5):379-380

58. Hannah RS, Roth SH, Chronic exposure to low concentrations of hydrogen sulfide produces abnormal growth in developing cerebella Purkinje cells

Department of Anatomy, University of Calgary, Alta, Canada

Neurosci Lett 1991 Jan 28; 122(2):225-228

59. Warenycia MW, Smith KA, Blashko CS, Kombian SB, Reiffenstien RJ, Monoamine oxidize inhibition as a sequel of hydrogen sulfide intoxication: increases in brain catecholamine and 5-hydroxytryptamine levels

Department of Pharmacology, University of Alberta, Edmonton, Canada

Arch Toxicol 1989; 63(2):131-136

60. Greer JJ, Reiffenstein RJ, Almedia AF, Carter JE, Sulfide-induced perturbations of the neuronal mechanisms controlling breathing in rats

Department of Physiology, University of Alberta, Edmonton, Canada

Skrajny B, Reiffenstein RJ, Sainsbury RS, Roth HS, Effects of repeated exposures of hydrogen sulfide on rat hippocampal EEG.

University of Calgary, Department of Pharmacology and Therapeutics, Calgary, Alberta, Canada

Toxicol Lett 1996 Jan; 84(1):43-53

61. Skrajny B, Hannah RS, Roth SH, Low concentrations of hydrogen sulfide alter monoamine levels in the developing rat central nervous system

Department of Pharmacology and Therapeutics, Faculty of Medicine, University of Calgary, Alta, Canada

Can J Physiol Pharmacol 1992 Nov; 70(11):1515-1518

62. Persson S, Edlund MB, Claesson R, Carlsson J, The formation of hydrogen sulfide and methyl mercaptan by oral bacteria

Department of Oral Microbiology, University of Umiea, Sweden

Oral Microbiol Immunol, 1990 Aug; 5(4):195-201

63. Claesson R, Edlund MB, Persson S, Carlsson J, Production of volatile sulfur compounds by various fusobacterium species

Department of Oral Microbiology, University of Umiea, Sweden

Oral Microbiol Immunol, 1990 Jun; 5(3):137-142

64. Finkelstein A, Benevenga NJ, The effect of methanethiol and methionine toxicity on the activities of cytochrome c oxidize and enzymes involved in protection from peroxidative damage

J Nutr 1986 Feb; 116(2):204-215

65. Mattila KJ, Valtonen VV, Nieminen M, Huttunen JK, Dental infection and the risk of new coronary events: prospective study of patients with documented coronary artery disease

First Department of Medicine, Helsinki University Central Hospital, Finland

Clin Infect Dis 1995 Mar; 20(3):588-592

66. Nord CE, Heimdahl A, Cardiovascular infections: bacterial endocarditis of oral origin. Pathogenesis and prophylaxis

Department of Microbiology, Huddinge University Hospital, Karolinska Institute, Stockholm, Sweden

J Clin Periodontol 1990 Aug; 17(7 Pt 2):494-496

67. Verhaaren H, Claeys G, Verschraegen G, de Niel C, Leroy J, Clement D, Endocarditis from a dental focus. Importance of oral hygiene in valve heart disease

68. Department of Pediatrics, University Hospital, Gent State University, Belgium

Int J Cardiol 1989 Jun; 23(3):343-347

Chapter 14: Understanding Energy for Good Health

1. You Are What You Ate by Sherry Rogers.

2. Robert Becker, *Cross Currents*

3. Robert Becker, *The Body Electric*

4. Janet G. Travell, M.D., *Myofascial Pain and Dysfunction (The Trigger Point Manual)* 1993, Waverly Press, Inc.

5. Vincent J. Speckhart, M.D., An *Electrodermal Analysis of Biological Conductance*, Biological Conductance Inc. 1340-1272 N. Great Neck Road, Box 188 - Virginia Beach VA 23453 USA

6. Summers AO., et al., Mercury released from dental "silver" fillings increases the incidence of multiply resistant bacteria in the oral and intestinal normal flora.

1991 Annual Meeting, American Society For Microbiology. Dallas, TX May 5-9, 1991. Abstract A137.

7. Summers AO; Wireman J; Vimy MJ; Lorscheider FL; Marshall B; Levy SB; Bennett S; Billiard L. Mercury released from dental "silver" fillings provokes an increase in mercury and antibiotic resistant bacteria in the primate oral and intestinal flora.

Antimicrobial Agents & Chemotherapy, 37:825-834, 1993.

8. Case Histories: Personal experience and results from patients treated.

Chapter 15: Taking Responsibility For Your health

1. Sherry Rogers, M.D. *Detoxify or Die*, 2002, Sand Key Company, Inc. 800-846-6687 www.prestigepublishing.com ISBN 1-887202-04-8

2. Sherry Rogers, M.D. *The High Blood Pressure Hoax*, 2005, Sand Key Company, Inc. 800-846-6687 www.prestigepublishing.com ISBN 1887202-05-6

3. Bremmer, D.K., *The Story of Dentistry* (3rd ed.), 1954. Dental Items of Interest Publishing Co., Inc. Brooklyn, NY.

4. ADA News. Editorial and accompanying patient handout on the safety of dental amalgam. Jan. 2, 1984.

5. ADA pamphlet Number W186. Dental amalgam filling dental health care needs. 1985.

6. When your patients ask about dental amalgam. JADA 122, August 1991.

7. Pleva J. Mercury from dental amalgams; exposure and effects. Int J Risk and Safety in Med. 3:1-22, 1992.

8. Council on Dental Materials, Instruments, and Equipment. Recommendations in dental mercury hygiene, 1984. JADA. 109:617-719, October 1984.

9. Svare, C.W. Dental amalgam related mercury vapor exposure. Cal Dent Assoc J. pp 55-60, Oct. 1984.

10. Vimy, M.J. and Lorscheider, f.L. Intra-oral air mercury released from dental amalgam. J.Dent Res. Vol 64:1069-1071, August 1985.

11. Vimy M.J. and Lorscheider, F.L. Intra-oral air mercury: estimation of daily dose from dental amalgam. J. Dent. Res. Vol 65:1072-1075, August 1985

12. Emler B.F. and Cardone M. Sr. An assessment of mercury in mouth air. J. Dent Res. Vol 64:247, IADR Abstract No. 652, 1985.

13. Patterson J.E., Weissberg B.G. and Dennison P.J. Mercury in the human breath from dental amalgams. Bull. Eviron Contam Toxicol. 34:459-468, 1985.

14. IPCs (international Programme on Chemical Safety) Environmental Health Criteria 118 Inorganic Mercury. Page 36, 1991. Published under the joint sponsorship of the United Nations Environment Programme, the International Labor Organization, and the World Health Organization.

15. Aposhian HV; Bruce DC; Alter W; Dart RC; Hurlbut KM: and Aposhian MM. Urinary mercury after administration of 2,3-dimercaptopropane-1-sulfonic acid: correlation with dental amalgam score. FaseB J> 6:2472, 1992.

16. Xander D; Ewers U; FreierI; Brockhaus. Studies on human exposure to mercury. 3 DMPS induced mobilization of mercury in subjects with and without amalgam fillings. Zentralblatt fur Hygiene und Umwelmedizin 192(5):447-454, Feb 1992.

17. Skare I. (Swedish National Board of Occupational Safety and Health). Mercury exposure from amalgam - a background study. Abstr Scand Occup Hyg Mtg. Iceland. Aug 1987.

18. Skare I and Egvist A. Amalgam restorations - an important source to human exposure of mercury and silver. LAKARTIDNINGEN 15:1299-1301, 1992.

19. WHO task group on evaluation of certain food additives and contaminants. Geneva: world Health Organization, 1972. (WHO Technical Report Series No 505).

20. Stock A and Curuel f. Der Quechsibergtehalt Der Menschichen Ausscheidumgn und des menschichen Blutes. Z Angew Chemie 47:641-647, 1934.

21. Frykjolm KO. Mercury from dental amalgam. UPPsala: Almquist & Wiskell, 1957.

22. Stortebecker P. *Mercury Poisoning from Dental Amalgams - Hazard to Human Brain*. Page 32-43, 1985. Bio-Probe, Inc. P.O. Box 608010, Orlando, FL 32860-8010.

23. Summers AO., et al. Mercury released from dental "silver" fillings increases the incidence of multiply resistant bacteria in the oral and intestinal normal flora. 1991 Annual Meeting, American Society for Microbiology. Dallas TX May 5-9, 1991 Abstract A137.

24. Schriever W. and Diamond L.E., Electromotive forces and electric currents caused by metallic dental fillings. J Dent Res. Vol 3 (2):205-228, 1952.

25. Schneider PE, Sarker NK. Mercury release from disperse alloy amalgam. JADA Abstract #630, 1982.

26. Hyams B.L. and Ballon H.C. Dissimilar metals in the mouth as a possible cause of otherwise unexplainable symptoms. Can Med Assoc J. Vol. XXIXX: 488-491, 1933.

27. Phillips R.W. *Skinner's Science of Dental Materials*. (7th edition) W.B. Saunders Co Philadelphia, 1973.

28. MIDR Workshop Biocompatibility of metals in dentistry. JADA Vol 109(3): 469-471, 1984.

29. Viola PL and Cassano GB., The effect of chlorine on mercury vapor intoxication. Auoradiographic Study. Med. Lavoro 59:437-444, 1968.

30. Cremer F. (ED.), Die Fabrkation De Silber-und Quecksilber-Spiegel. Hartlebens Verl., Wien u. Leipzig 1904.

31. Viola PL. L'influenza del cloro sull'introssicazinoe da vapori di mercurio. Med Lavoro 58; 60-65, 1967.

31. Djerassi E. and Berova N. The possibilities of allergic reaction from silver amalgam restorations. Int Dent J. 19(4):481-488, 1969.

32. Miller E.G., Perry W.L. and Wagner M.J, Prevalence of mercury hyper sensitivity in dental students. J Prosthetic Dent. 58(2):235-237, Aug 1987.

33. ADA. When your patients ask about mercury in amalgam. JADA. 120:395-8. April 1990.

34. Schiele R. et al. Studies on the mercury content in brain and kidney related to number and condition of amalgam fillings. Inst Occup & Social Med. Univ Erlangen-Nurnberrg. Symosium March 12 1984, cologne. Amalgam-Viepoints fro Medicine and Dental Medicine.

35. Friberg L. et al. Mercury in the central nervous system in relation to amalgam fillings. LAKARTIDNINGEN 83(7):519-522, 1986.

36. Eggleston D.W. and Nylander M. Correlation of dental amalgam with mercury in brain tissue. J Prosthetic Dent. 58(7):519-522, 1986.

37. Hanson M. Mercury Bibliography (3rd Edition) 285 symptoms of mercury toxicity and 12000 mercury citations. Bio-Probe, Inc. P.O. Box 608010 Orlando FL 32860-8010.

38. Wenstrup D; ehmann WD; and Markesberry WR. Trace element imbalances in isolated subcellular fractions of Alzheimer's disease brains. Brain Research, 533:125-131, 1990.

39. Duhr E; Pendergrass C; Kasarkis J; Slevin J; and haley B. Hg2+ induces GTP-Tubulin interactions in rat brain similar to those observed in Alzheimer's disease. FASEB, 75th Annual Meeting, April 21-25, 1991 Atlanta, Georgia, Abstract 493.

40. The Alzheimer's Disease Research Center Update Newsletter, Fall 1991 University of Kentucky, Lexington, Kentucky.

31. Clarkson T.W., Rriberg L., Hursh J.B. and Nylander M. The prediction of intake of mercury vapor from amalgams. In: Biological Monitoring of Toxic Metals. Plenum Press, NY, 1988.

42. DENTAL AMALGAM: A scientific review and recommended Public Health Service Strategy for research, education and regulation. January 1993, Department of Health and Human Services, Public Health Service.

43. Hahn, LJ; Kloiber, R; Takahashi, Y; Vimy, MJ; Loscheider, Fl. Dental "silver" fillings: a source of mercury exposure revealed by whole-body image scan and tissue analysis. FASEB j. 3:2641-6. Dec 1989.

44. Vimy, MJ; Takahashi, Y; Lorscheider, FI. Maternal-fetal distribution of mercury (203 Hg) released from dental amalgam fillings. Amer J Physiol. 258:R939-45. April 1990.

45. Danscher G; Horsted-Bindley P; and Rungby J. Traces of mercury in organs from primates with amalgam fillings. Exp Molecular Path 52:291-299, 1990.

46. Hahn LJ; Kloiber R; Leininger RW; Vimy MJ; and Lorscheider FL. Whole-Body imaging of the distribution of mercury released from dental fillings into monkey tissues. FASEB J 4:3256-3260, 1990.

Chapter 16: Dental Materials Are One of the Keys to Health.

See Chapter 15 references.

Chapter 17: X-Rays

1. Bhaskar, SN: Periapical lesion-types., incidence and clinical features. Oral Surg 1966, 21:659

2. George Meinig, D.D.S., F.A.C.D. *Root Canal Cover-up Exposed!* X-rays on Pages: 20, 37, 38, 39, 40, 48, 53, 57, 76, 78, 90, 121, 124, 129, 136, 172,

Chapter 18: Finding A Suitable Holistic Dentist

Chapter 19: Computerized Electro-dermal Screening

Contact the following for literature:

1. Orion Service and Support 1219 South 1840 West, Orem, UT 84058

Phone: 801-226-6745

2. Synergy Health Systems 1223 Wilshire Blvd #321 Santa Monica CA

Phone: 310-394-6497

3. Vibrant Health Steven Edmond 888-53601294

Chapter 20: Body Health Dentistry

1. Vimy, MJ; Takahashi, Y; Lorscheider, FI. Maternal-fetal distribution of mercury (203 Hg) released from dental amalgam fillings. Amer J Physiol. 258:R939-45. April 1990.

2. Summers AO., et al. Mercury released from dental "silver" fillings increases the incidence of multiply resistant bacteria in the oral and intestinal normal flora. 1991 Annual Meeting, American Society for Microbiology. Dallas TX May 5-9, 1991 Abstract A137.

3. Vimy MJ; Hahn LJ; Kloiber R; Leininger RW; Lorscheider FL.Whole body imaging of the distribution of mercury released from dental fillings into monkey tissues. FASEB J 4:3256-3260, 1990

4. Vimy MJ; Summers AO; Wireman J; Lorscheider FL; Marshall B; Levy SB; Bennett S; Billiard L. Mercury released from dental "silver" fillings provokes an increase in mercury and antibiotic resistant bacteria in the primate oral and intestinal flora. Antimicrobial Agents & Chemotherapy, 37:825-834, 1993.

Chapter 21: Electrodermal Screening Health Professional Start Here

1. Vimy MJ; Hahn LJ; Kloiber R; Leininger RW; Lorscheider FL, Whole body imaging of the distribution of mercury released from dental fillings into monkey tissues.

FASEB J 4:3256-3260, 1990

2. Vimy MJ, Summers AO, Wireman J, Lorscheider FL, Marshall B, Levy SB, Bennett S, Billiard L, Mercury released from dental "silver" fillings provokes an increase in mercury and antibiotic resistant bacteria in the primate oral and intestinal flora.

Antimicrobial Agents & Chemotherapy, 37:825-834, 1993.

Chapter 22: Dry Socket – Cause and Treatment

Dry socket medication introduced by I. L. Cook, DDS in 1921

Chapter 23: Build, Not Destroy, Your Practice

Dr. I. L. Cook, D.D.S., and Dr. D. L. Cook, D.D.S, personal experience.

Chapter 24: Environmental Dentistry (Instrumentation)

Chapter 25: Teeth and Body Energy Chart